Epilepsy Surgery: The Emerging Field of Neuromodulation

Guest Editors

EDWARD F. CHANG, MD
NICHOLAS M. BARBARO, MD

NEUROSURGERY CLINICS OF NORTH AMERICA

www.neurosurgery.theclinics.com

Consulting Editors
ANDREW T. PARSA, MD, PhD
PAUL C. McCORMICK, MD, MPH

October 2011 • Volume 22 • Number 4

SAUNDERS an imprint of ELSEVIER, Inc.

W.B. SAUNDERS COMPANY
A Division of Elsevier Inc.

1600 John F. Kennedy Blvd. • Suite 1800 • Philadelphia, PA 19103-2899

http://www.theclinics.com

NEUROSURGERY CLINICS OF NORTH AMERICA Volume 22, Number 4
October 2011 ISSN 1042-3680, ISBN-13: 978-1-4557-1028-7

Editor: Jessica McCool
Developmental Editor: Donald Mumford

Neurosurgery Clinics of North America (ISSN 1042-3680) is published quarterly by Elsevier Inc., 360 Park Avenue South, New York, NY 10010-1710. Months of issue are January, April, July, and October. Business and Editorial Offices: 1600 John F. Kennedy Blvd., Suite 1800, Philadelphia, PA 19103-2899. Customer Service Office: 11830 Westline Industrial Drive, St. Louis, MO 63146. Periodicals postage paid at New York, NY, and additional mailing offices. Subscription prices are $317.00 per year (US individuals), $492.00 per year (US institutions), $347.00 per year (Canadian individuals), $601.00 per year (Canadian institutions), $443.00 per year (international individuals), $601.00 per year (international institutions), $156.00 per year (US students), and $214.00 per year (international students). International air speed delivery is included in all *Clinics* subscription prices. All prices are subject to change without notice. **POSTMASTER:** Send address changes to *Neurosurgery Clinics of North America*, Elsevier Periodicals Customer Service, 11830 Westline Industrial Drive, St. Louis, MO 63146. **Customer Service: 1-800-654-2452 (US and Canada). From outside the US and Canada, call: 1-314-453-7041. Fax: 1-314-453-5170. E-mail: JournalsCustomerService-usa@elsevier.com (for print support) and journalsonlinesupport-usa@elsevier.com (for online support).**

Reprints. For copies of 100 or more, of articles in this publication, please contact the Commercial Reprints Department, Elsevier Inc., 360 Park Avenue South, New York, NY 10010-1710. Tel. (212) 633-3812; Fax: (212) 462-1935; E-mail: reprints@elsevier.com.

Neurosurgery Clinics of North America is covered in *MEDLINE/PubMed (Index Medicus), EMBASE/Excerpta Medica, and Current Contents/Clinical Medicine (CC/CM).*

Printed and bound by CPI Group (UK) Ltd, Croydon, CR0 4YY

Transferred to Digital Print 2011

Contributors

CONSULTING EDITORS

ANDREW T. PARSA, MD, PhD
Associate Professor, Principal Investigator,
Brain Tumor Research Center, Reza and
Georgianna Khatib Endowed Chair in Skull
Base Tumor Surgery, Department of
Neurological Surgery, University of California,
San Francisco, San Francisco, California

PAUL C. McCORMICK, MD, MPH, FACS
Herbert & Linda Gallen Professor of
Neurological Surgery, Department of
Neurological Surgery, Columbia University
Medical Center, New York, New York

GUEST EDITORS

EDWARD F. CHANG, MD
Assistant Professor, Departments of
Neurological Surgery and Physiology,
University of California, San Francisco,
San Francisco, California

NICHOLAS M. BARBARO, MD
Professor, Departments of Neurological
Surgery and Physiology, University of
California, San Francisco, San Francisco,
California

AUTHORS

KURTIS I. AUGUSTE, MD
Department of Neurological Surgery,
Epilepsy Center, University of California,
San Francisco, San Francisco, California

EDWARD F. CHANG, MD
Assistant Professor, Departments of
Neurological Surgery and Physiology,
University of California, San Francisco,
San Francisco, California

IAN A. COOK, MD
Depression Research and Clinic Program,
Semel Institute for Neuroscience and Human
Behavior at UCLA, Los Angeles, California

CHRISTOPHER M. DEGIORGIO, MD, FAAN
Department of Neurology, David Geffen School
of Medicine at UCLA, Los Angeles, California

SHARANYA ARCOT DESAI, BE, MSc
Department of Neurosurgery, Emory University
School of Medicine; Laboratory for
Neuroengineering, Georgia Institute of
Technology, Atlanta, Georgia

DARIO J. ENGLOT, MD, PhD
Department of Neurological Surgery, Epilepsy
Center, University of California, San Francisco,
San Francisco, California

ERIKA E. FANSELOW, PhD
Department of Neurobiology, University of
Pittsburgh School of Medicine, Pittsburgh,
Pennsylvania

KOSTAS N. FOUNTAS, MD, PhD
Assistant Professor of Neurosurgery,
Department of Neurosurgery, University
Hospital of Larisa, School of Medicine,
University of Thessaly, Biopolis, Larissa,
Greece

PAUL R. GIGANTE, MD
Department of Neurological Surgery, Columbia
University, New York, New York

ROBERT R. GOODMAN, MD, PhD
Associate Professor, Department of
Neurological Surgery, Columbia University;
Chairman, Department of Neurological
Surgery, St Luke's-Roosevelt, New York,
New York

ROBERT E. GROSS, MD, PhD
Departments of Neurosurgery and Neurology, Emory University School of Medicine; Coulter Department of Biomedical Engineering, Georgia Institute of Technology, Atlanta, Georgia

YU HAN, MS
Department of Electrical Engineering, University of California, Santa Cruz, Santa Cruz, California

TOMOR HARNOD, MD, PhD
Department of Neurosurgery, Hualein Tzu Chi Medical Center, Hualein, Taiwan

YUE-LOONG HSIN, MD
Director of Epilepsy Center, Chair of Neurology, Department of Neurology, Hualien Tzu Chi Medical Center, Hualein, Taiwan

LEON D. IASEMIDIS, PhD
Associate Professor, Harrington Department of Biomedical Engineering, School of Biological and Health Systems Engineering, Arizona State University; Affiliate Professor, Department of Electrical Engineering, School of Electrical, Computer and Energy Engineering, Arizona State University, Tempe; Adjunct Professor, Department of Neurology, Mayo Clinic, Phoenix, Arizona

NEALEN G. LAXPATI, BS
Department of Neurosurgery, Emory University School of Medicine; Coulter Department of Biomedical Engineering, Georgia Institute of Technology, Atlanta, Georgia

WENTAI LIU, PhD
Campus Director of NSF-ERC on Biomimetic MicroElectronic Systems, Professor of Electrical Engineering, Department of Electrical Engineering, University of California, Santa Cruz, Santa Cruz, California

YINN CHER OOI, BS
Jefferson Medical College, Thomas Jefferson University Hospital, Philadelphia, Pennsylvania

JOHN D. ROLSTON, MD, PhD
Department of Neurological Surgery, University of California, San Francisco, San Francisco, California

STEVEN M. ROTHMAN, MD
Professor of Neurology, Department of Neurology, University of Minnesota Medical School, Minneapolis, Minnesota

LARA M. SCHRADER, MD
Department of Neurology, David Geffen School of Medicine at UCLA, Los Angeles, California

ASHWINI SHARAN, MD, FACS
Department of Neurosurgery, Thomas Jefferson University Hospital, Philadelphia, Pennsylvania

MATTHEW D. SMYTH, MD
Associate Professor of Neurosurgery and Pediatrics, Department of Neurosurgery, Washington University, St Louis, Missouri

VIKAAS S. SOHAL, MD, PhD
Department of Psychiatry; Keck Center for Integrative Neuroscience; Sloan-Swartz Center for Theoretical Neurobiology, University of California, San Francisco, San Francisco, California

JOHN C. STYLIARAS, MD
Department of Neurosurgery, Thomas Jefferson University Hospital, Philadelphia, Pennsylvania

FELICE T. SUN, PhD
NeuroPace, Inc, Mountain View, California

JOSE F. TELLEZ-ZENTENO, MD, PhD
Associate Professor, Division of Neurology, Department of Medicine, University of Saskatchewan, Saskatoon, Saskatchewan, Canada

SAMUEL WIEBE, MD
Professor, Department of Clinical Neurosciences, University of Calgary, Calgary, Alberta, Canada

Contents

Direct electrical stimulation of the brain is an increasingly popular means of treating refractory epilepsy. Although there has been moderate success in human trials, the rate of seizure freedom does not yet compare favorably to resective surgery. It therefore remains critical to advance experimental investigations aimed toward understanding brain stimulation and its utility. This article introduces the concepts necessary for understanding these experimental studies, describing recording and stimulation technology, animal models of epilepsy, and various subcortical targets of stimulation. Bidirectional and closed-loop device technologies are also highlighted, along with the challenges presented by their experimental use.

Medically refractory epilepsy is a morbid condition, and many patients are poor candidates for surgical resection because of multifocal seizure origin or eloquence near epileptic foci. Vagus nerve stimulation (VNS) was approved in 1997 by the US Food and Drug Administration as an adjunctive treatment of intractable epilepsy for individuals aged 12 years and more with partial epilepsy. Controversy persists regarding the efficacy of VNS for epilepsy and about which patient populations respond best to therapy. In this article, the authors retrospectively studied a patient outcome registry and report the largest, to their knowledge, analysis of VNS outcomes in epilepsy.

The unique ability to stimulate bilaterally, extracranially, and non-invasively may represent a significant advantage to invasive neuromodulation therapies. In humans thus far the technique has been applied noninvasively, and is termed external trigeminal nerve stimulation (eTNSTM).

With the growing applications for deep brain stimulators (DBS) in recent years, interest in using DBS as an option for patients with epilepsy has increased. Thalamic DBS appears to be a viable minimally invasive treatment for patients experiencing medically intractable seizures. Thalamic DBS has been associated with significant reduction in seizure frequency and an improvement in overall quality of life, especially in patients who have failed maximal antiepileptic drugs or other surgical alternatives. However, further work is necessary to identify the subgroups of patients experiencing medically intractable seizures who may benefit from DBS, and also to indentify optimal stimulation parameters and mode of stimulation.

Neuromodulation is one of the fastest growing fields in neurosurgery, as reflected by the growing interest in the use of electrical brain stimulation (EBS) to treat drug-resistant epilepsy, pain, and movement disorders. Hippocampal stimulation should be regarded as an experimental therapy for epilepsy, and patients considered for this intervention should do so in the context of a well-designed randomized controlled trial. Only well-conducted, blinded, randomized trials, followed by long-term systematic observation will yield a clear picture of the effect of this promising therapy, and will help guide its future use. This article provides a critical review of the best available evidence on hippocampal stimulation for epilepsy.

Neurostimulation in epilepsy has witnessed a century-long evolution that has resulted in the use of neurostimulation to both modulate and suppress abnormal neuronal firing. The recent development of advanced responsive stimulation via a closed-loop device (the RNS System) has provided evidence that surgical epilepsy treatment continues to move toward the possibility of reducing or eliminating seizures in medically refractory patients.

Deep brain stimulation (DBS) is an established treatment for Parkinson's disease, and is increasingly used for other neuropsychiatric conditions including epilepsy. Nevertheless, neural mechanisms for DBS and other forms of neurostimulation remain elusive. The authors measured effects of responsive neurostimulation on intracranially recorded activity from participants in a clinical investigation to assess the safety of an implantable responsive neurostimulation system in epilepsy (RNS™ System, NeuroPace, Inc.). Neurostimulation acutely suppressed gamma frequency (35–100 Hz) phase-locking. This may represent a therapeutic mechanism by which responsive neurostimulation can suppress epileptiform activity and disconnect stimulated regions from downstream targets in epilepsy and other neuropsychiatric conditions.

Epilepsy is characterized by intermittent, paroxysmal, hypersynchronous electrical activity that may remain localized and/or spread and severely disrupt the brain's normal multitask and multiprocessing function. Epileptic seizures are the hallmarks of such activity. The ability to issue warnings in real time of impending seizures may lead to novel diagnostic tools and treatments for epilepsy. Applications may range from a warning to the patient to avert seizure-associated injuries, to automatic timely administration of an appropriate stimulus. Seizure prediction could become an integral part of the treatment of epilepsy through neuromodulation, especially in the new generation of closed-loop seizure control systems.

Yu Han, Yue-Loong Hsin, Tomor Harnod, and Wentai Liu

Many factors underlying basic epileptic conditions determine the characteristics of epileptic seizures and the therapeutic outcome. Diagnosis and treatment rely on the clinical manifestations as well as electroencephalographic (EEG) epileptic activities. This article briefly reviews the fundamentals of the EEG, interictal, and ictal electrical activities of both extracranial and intracranial EEG of partial epilepsies, based on the information obtained from epilepsy patients who have undergone epilepsy surgery. The authors also present the status of their current research, focusing on decomposed seizure sources and the rendered spatial-temporal transitions in focal seizure.

Kostas N. Fountas

Invasive electroencephalography via subdural implanted electrodes is essential for the identification and localization of the epileptogenic focus in a large percentage of cases of medically refractory epilepsy. The implantation of subdural electrodes constitutes a widely used method for the preoperative investigation of these patients. However, their implantation has been associated with the occurrence of some rare but potentially serious complications. This article systematically reviews the literature regarding safety issues, potential complications, and complication avoidance strategies associated with the implantation of subdural electrodes. Knowledge of all the reported complications may help in their early detection and their prompt management.

Matthew D. Smyth and Steven M. Rothman

Focal cooling may provide a safe, nondestructive alternative to resective and disconnective strategies that have been proposed or used to control refractory epilepsy. Observations of the effects of direct application of iced saline on the cortical surface during cortical mapping surgery and induced seizures have led to interest in developing implantable cooling therapy devices for refractory localizable epilepsies. In this article, the authors provide an overview of the historical background, physiology, and animal and human data leading to the development of implantable cooling devices for the treatment of medically refractory epilepsy.

Neurosurgery Clinics of North America

RELATED INTEREST

Emergency Medicine Clinics, February 2011 (Volume 29, Issue 1)
Seizures
Andy Jagoda, MD, and Edward P. Sloan, MD, MPH, *Guest Editors*
http://www.emed.theclinics.com/

VISIT THE CLINICS ONLINE!

Access your subscription at:
www.theclinics.com

Preface

Epilepsy Surgery: The Emerging Field of Neuromodulation

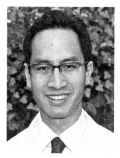
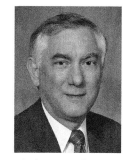

Edward F. Chang, MD   Nicholas M. Barbaro, MD
Guest Editors

Epilepsy is a devastating neurological disorder that afflicts nearly 1% of the population. While resective surgery has been demonstrated to have excellent seizure-control outcomes in selected patients, many others are not candidates because the epileptogenic zone is multifocal and/or includes eloquent brain regions. Furthermore, resective surgery can be associated with neurocognitive effects, which are sometimes irreversible.

Over the last 30 years, tremendous progress has been made in expanding non-resective approaches to epilepsy surgery. With new advances in seizure detection, signal processing, and electrical stimulation, there is significant interest in developing a new generation of implantable devices for patients with intractable seizure disorders.

In this issue, we focus on emerging device technology in the field of epilepsy surgery. The articles are a compilation of topics that are highly relevant to neural interface technology. We are pleased to have significant contributions from experts in engineering, neurology, basic neuroscience, and neurosurgery. Together, they address the theoretical background, recent advances in research, and clinical outcomes of current and future devices in epilepsy surgery.

To start, Rolston and colleagues provide a comprehensive in-depth review of progress and obstacles in recording and stimulation technology applied to epilepsy. Several structures of the nervous system have been proposed as potential targets of device-based neuromodulation. Currently, the only FDA-approved device for epilepsy is the Vagal Nerve Stimulation by Cyberonics, Inc. Englot and coworkers report the largest analysis of VNS outcomes and their predictors performed to date from thousands of patients in the Cyberonics registry.

As a promising alternative to the extracranial-based device, DeGiorgio and colleagues report the development of infraorbital or supraorbital trigeminal nerve stimulation. This new approach offers the possibility of testing efficacy percutaneously before implantation.

The majority of other devices involve direct intracranial stimulation. Ooi and coworkers review the available literature on the anterior thalamus as a target for deep brain stimulation, including technical nuances and clinical results for this target. Tellez-Zenteno and Wiebe present a critical review of the emerging evidence for hippocampal stimulation as well as outlining what outstanding questions remain for prospective trials of efficacy.

Closed-loop systems that detect seizures to then trigger electrical stimulation to abort them are making clinical progress. Gigante and Goodman provide a historical overview and report on recent clinical trials conducted for the Responsive

doi:10.1016/j.nec.2011.07.012

neurosurgery.theclinics.com

Neurostimulation System (RNS) from Neuropace. How cortical stimulation reduces seizures is unclear. Sohal and Sun report novel mechanistic findings from patients implanted with the RNS system, suggesting that stimulation acutely desynchronizes long-range gamma frequency activity, thereby functionally "disconnecting" the epileptogenic network.

Unpredictability is a major factor contributing to the morbidity and mortality related to seizures. Recent advances in seizure prediction research are leading to wide-ranging potential applications including systems that can warn patients of impending seizures or triggering stimulation in closed loop devices. Iasemidis presents an excellent review of how a dynamical systems approach applied to epilepsy has led to a better understanding of seizure onsets, periods of susceptibility, and localization. Han and colleagues report on the powerful application of independent components analysis for improving the reliability and robustness of seizure detection and localization.

For intracranial devices, subdural or depth electrodes are the most common interface with the brain parenchyma. Fountas performed a systematic review of the literature to report the safety and complication avoidance associated with chronic indwelling electrodes.

Finally, Smyth and Rothman describe a completely alternative approach using focal cortical cooling. They present an overview of the rationale and preclinical data in animals and humans leading to the development of implantable cooling devices.

The field of neuromodulation for epilepsy is in its infancy, and significant knowledge gaps remain regarding how best to apply rapidly developing technology to achieve the best clinical outcomes. This issue is intended to stimulate further efforts in innovative uses of technology to suppress seizures without inducing unwanted side effects.

Edward F. Chang, MD
Nicholas M. Barbaro, MD

Departments of Neurological Surgery
and Physiology
University of California, San Francisco
505 Parnassus Avenue, Room M779
San Francisco, CA 94143-0112, USA

E-mail addresses:
ChangEd@neurosurg.ucsf.edu (E.F. Chang)
barbaron@neurosurg.ucsf.edu (N.M. Barbaro)

Electrical Stimulation for Epilepsy: Experimental Approaches

John D. Rolston, MD, PhD[a], Sharanya Arcot Desai, BE, MSc[b,c],
Nealen G. Laxpati, BS[b,d], Robert E. Gross, MD, PhD[b,d,e],*

KEYWORDS

- Brain electrical stimulation • Epilepsy
- Animal models of epilepsy
- Recording and stimulation technology

Direct electrical stimulation of the brain is an increasingly popular means of treating refractory epilepsy.[1] Although there has been moderate success in human trials, the rate of seizure freedom does not yet compare favorably to resective surgery.[1] It therefore remains critical to advance experimental investigations aimed toward understanding brain stimulation and its utility. This article introduces the concepts necessary for understanding these experimental studies, describing recording and stimulation technology, animal models of epilepsy, and the various subcortical targets of stimulation that have been investigated. Because of the continued interest in bidirectional and closed-loop devices, these technologies are also highlighted, along with the challenges presented by their experimental use.[2]

ELECTRODE RECORDING
Types of Signals

Depending on the properties of the recording electronics (electrode material, size, position, sampling rate of the analog-to-digital converters, and so forth), signals ranging from individual action potentials to the electrocorticogram can be recorded, with each type of signal providing a different scale of information about brain physiology.

Single units

When a neuron generates an action potential (AP), the current across its cell membrane generates a complex electric field. An electrode placed in this external electric field will detect this activity, referred to as a *spike*. Recording such spiking activity from individual neurons is known as *single unit* recording. Unlike intracellularly recorded APs, which are commonly recorded using patch-clamp techniques, extracellular spikes vary markedly in morphology and even polarity, and are dependent on the geometry of the cell and the location of the recording electrode. Although these variations may be of interest, in that they may indicate location of the recording electrode in well-defined neural tissue,[3] most investigations instead examine evoked spikes or characteristics of spike

[a] Department of Neurological Surgery, University of California at San Francisco, 505 Parnassus Avenue, Room 779M, San Francisco, CA 94143, USA
[b] Department of Neurosurgery, Emory University School of Medicine, 1365-B Clifton Road Suite 2200, Atlanta, GA 30322, USA
[c] Laboratory for Neuroengineering, Georgia Institute of Technology, 313 Ferst Drive, Atlanta, GA 30332, USA
[d] Coulter Department of Biomedical Engineering, Georgia Institute of Technology, 313 Ferst Drive, Atlanta, GA 30332, USA
[e] Department of Neurology, Emory University School of Medicine, 101 Woodruff Circle, Atlanta, GA 30322, USA
* Corresponding author. Department of Neurosurgery, Emory University School of Medicine, 1365-B Clifton Road Suite 2200, Atlanta, GA 30322.
E-mail address: rgross@emory.edu

Neurosurg Clin N Am 22 (2011) 425–442
doi:10.1016/j.nec.2011.07.010
1042-3680/11/$ – see front matter © 2011 Elsevier Inc. All rights reserved.

trains. Microelectrodes with a tip diameter on the order of micrometers and geometric surface area less than 2000 to 4000 μm^2 are commonly used for recording the extracellular activity of single neurons.[4] The extracellularly recorded action potential is typically less than 100 μV, about 2 orders of magnitude lower than that of a corresponding intracellular recording.

During single-unit recordings, the largest component of signal noise arises from the multitude of undifferentiated background action potentials and synaptic potentials (neural noise). However, electrode impedance also contributes and is known as thermal noise, with higher impedance electrodes consequently demonstrating more noise and a lower signal-to-noise ratio. In addition, high electrode impedance in combination with the distributed capacitance between the electrode and the recording amplifier will reduce the electrodes' high-frequency response.[4] One method of improving the signal-to-noise ratio is to reduce electrode impedance without increasing the surface extent of the electrodes. This can be achieved either through sputtering or electroplating the tip with a biocompatible material that reduces the impedance without increasing the surface extent of the electrodes.[5]

Multiunit activity

If activity from more than one single neuron is detected by a microelectrode, the resulting polyneuronal activity is often referred to as multiunit activity (MUA). Spike-sorting methods can then be used to putatively identify each recorded waveform as originating from a particular cell.[6] However, another definition of MUA relies on isolating the "neural noise" described previously. If the electrical activity above a certain frequency is isolated (eg, >300 Hz), the power of those high frequencies can be used as a surrogate for large-scale spiking activity from multiple neurons. This high-pass signal is then typically rectified and low-pass filtered to generate a time-varying estimate of MUA.[7]

Local field potentials

The local field potential (LFP) is the low-frequency (arbitrarily <300 Hz) summed synaptic activity recorded extracellularly from a population of neurons. It can be isolated from microelectrodes or macroelectrodes. Recent studies suggest that the LFP signal originates within a range of 250 μm from the recording electrode,[8] smaller than the previously reported range of 400 μm to a few millimeters.[9,10]

LFP recordings enable the visualization of prominent brain oscillations (eg, alpha, beta, theta,

gamma, delta) when electrodes are placed in appropriate regions. There is some debate about whether the various frequency components of the LFP have unique corresponding spatial footprints. For example, it has been proposed that the higher frequencies (in the gamma range, around 25–90 Hz) may carry information that is more local than the lower frequencies, perhaps as a result of the capacitive properties of neural tissue.[8,11]

Electrocorticography

Electrocorticography (ECoG) uses macroelectrodes (~5 mm in diameter) to record directly from the brain, either superficially or at depth. Although, as compared with electroencephalography (EEG), ECoG is invasive, it enables higher spatial resolution (ie, tenths of millimeters vs centimeters), broader bandwidth (ie, 0–200 Hz vs 0–40 Hz), and higher amplitude (ie, 50–100 μV maximum vs 10–20 μV). Surface ECoG does not require electrodes to penetrate the cortex, and thus may have greater long-term stability and safety compared with single-unit penetrating microelectrodes[12]; however, it lacks the spatial resolution of implanted microelectrode and macroelectrode recordings.

Electroencephalography

EEG refers to electrical recordings made with macro electrodes positioned noninvasively on the subject's scalp (but could include other approaches, eg, epidural peg electrodes). Standard montages are used (eg, the international 10–20 system), but are often supplanted by extra electrodes. EEG is most commonly used in the diagnosis and classification of epilepsy, with its main advantages being that it is noninvasive and inexpensive. However, EEG does have several limitations. Large areas of the cortex need to be activated synchronously to generate enough potential to be recorded extracranially. Propagation of electrical activity along physiologic pathways in extracellular spaces may give a misleading impression as to the source of the electrical activity. Furthermore, EEG suffers from poor spatial resolution, confounding seizure foci localization. Nevertheless, EEG continues to play a central role in the diagnosis of epilepsy and other neurologic disorders, and has been used extensively in conjunction with other diagnostic techniques.[13]

Types of Electrodes

According to Merrill and colleagues,[14] the ideal material for building electrodes should satisfy 6 requirements. It should (1) be biologically compatible,

(2) maintain its mechanical integrity during the surgical procedure, (3) have sufficient charge storage capacity, (4) not undergo electrochemical reactions that produce toxic products, (5) not undergo Faradaic corrosion reactions, and (6) be stable for the duration of the implant. Criterion (5) depends highly on the duration of implantation—electrodes used in acute studies are unlikely to fail because of corrosion. Based on their size, electrodes can be broadly classified into 2 categories: microelectrodes and macroelectrodes.

Microelectrodes

Microelectrodes are small-diameter (<50 μm) electrodes, typically used in the recording of single-unit activity. Depending on the material and diameter, their impedances range from tens of kΩ to more than tens of MΩ. In addition to recording, microelectrodes can be used to deliver stimulation. In a direct application of Ohm's law, the higher the impedance of the microelectrode, the higher the required voltage to deliver the same amount of current. Thus, microelectrode impedance plays a major role in determining the maximum stimulation potential that may be applied to the electrode without causing undesirable breakdown of water molecules into hydrogen and oxygen gas. This potential limit is known as the "water window," and with high impedance electrodes, care should be taken to ensure the stimulation potential does not exceed an acceptable range.[14] One way of circumventing this problem is to reduce the impedance of microelectrodes while maintaining their small surface extent, for example by electroplating their tips with a biocompatible material. The material deposited with electroplating, however, can sometimes be shed during long recordings, limiting the use of electroplating in chronic recordings. More recently it has been shown by our group that sonicoplating—electroplating under ultrasonic agitation—can significantly improve the durability of plating.[5] Lowering microelectrode impedance will produce additional advantages, such as reduced thermal noise, which increases as a function of the electrode impedance, and smaller stimulation artifacts. Reduction of stimulation artifact is particularly important for closed-loop applications, which are discussed later in this article.

Metal microelectrodes The performance of metal microelectrodes for neural recording and stimulation depends on their geometric, electrical, and mechanical properties.[15] The most frequently used metals for manufacturing microelectrodes include stainless steel, platinum, iridium, tungsten, titanium, nickel-chromium, and their alloys. Copper and silver are known to cause tissue necrosis and hence are not often used.[4] Electrodes are often covered in an insulating material—such as varnish, epoxy, parylene, glass, Teflon, or polyimide—to within a few micrometers of their tip, which is left exposed to record the highly localized extracellular potentials induced by currents in one or a few of the closest neurons. They may also be used to deliver highly localized stimulation.

Tetrodes can be made by twisting 4 microwires around each other and applying sufficient heat to bind them together by melting their insulation. The 4 microelectrode tips are then within a micrometer from each other, and consequently have a high probability of picking up APs simultaneously from the same neurons. The shape of the APs picked up by the 4 electrodes, although different (dependent on their location with respect to the firing neuron) is also very reproducible (they record the same shape of activity whenever that particular neuron fires), making spike sorting simple and reliable, using a process akin to triangulation to identify particular cells. The tetrode configuration additionally provides stability to the microwires during implantation.[16] Another common practice is to arrange multiple microwires onto a single shaft (microwire arrays) for recording and/or stimulating multiple single units at the same time. TDT (Achua, FL, USA), Neuronexus Technologies Inc (Ann Arbor, MI, USA), and Plexon (Dallas, TX, USA) are among the vendors who sell such microwire arrays for use in animal studies. More recently, Bartels and colleagues,[17] have designed neurotrophic electrodes for increasing the longevity and stability of recorded signals. Their design induces neurite growth into a glass cone that covers the tip of gold microelectrodes insulated with Teflon, anchoring the glass tip to the neuropil.

Other types of microelectrodes Silicone-based microelectrode arrays are gaining popularity as an alternative to microwire arrays. The most significant advantage of the silicon-based microelectrode technology is that it enables the monolithic integration of electronics, such as amplifiers, filters, and multiplexers, into the probe structure. These active microelectrodes improve the quality of recorded signals over passive microelectrode arrays (without integration of electronics).[18,19]

PDMS (polydimethylsiloxane)-based microelectrodes are deformable, enabling conformation to the structure from which they are recording and/or stimulating. Such flexible designs hold great promise for recording from structures that are otherwise inaccessible to the rigid metal/silicone-based microelectrodes, although they are not yet available for use in human subjects (**Fig. 1**).[20,21]

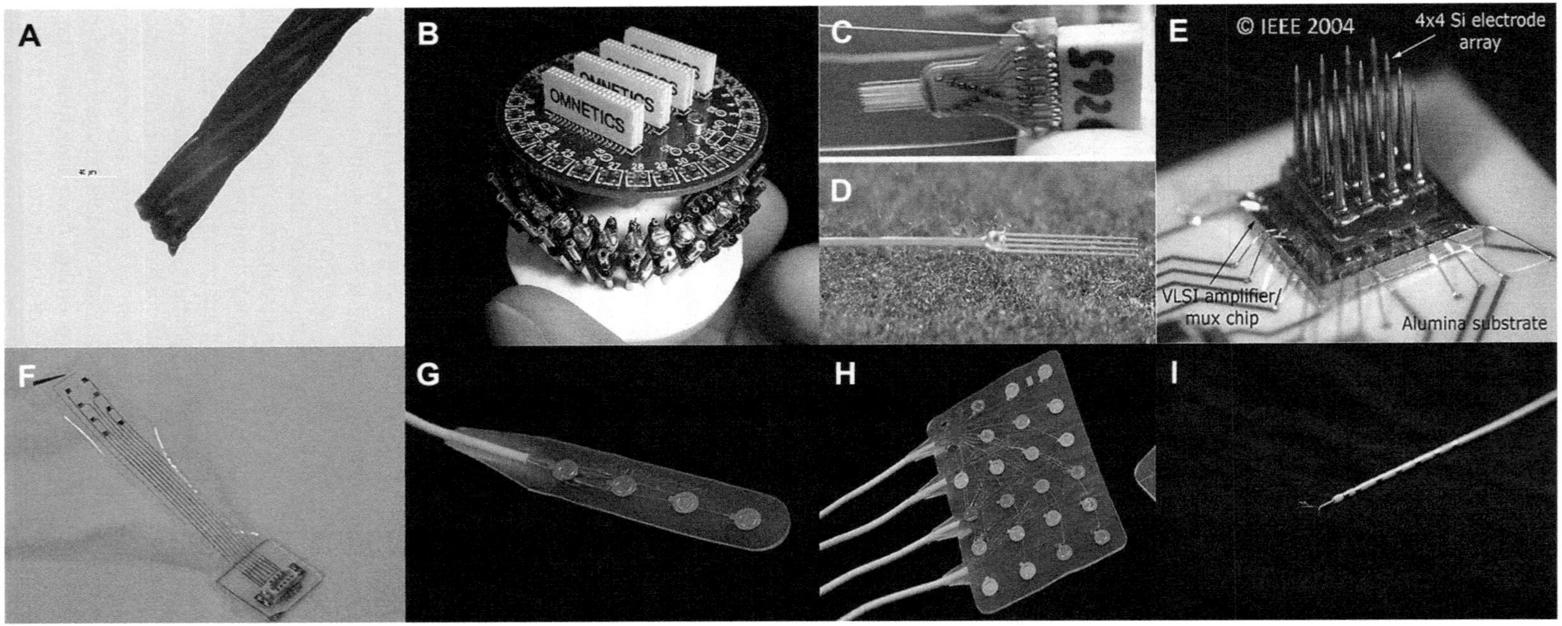

Fig. 1. (*A*) Tetrode: made by twisting 4 microwires around each other. Mainly used in single-unit recording for spike-sorting purposes. (*B*) An example of a recording headstage. This particular setup allows multiple tetrodes to be driven into the brain tissue. The individual screws in the headstage allow the experimenter to drive the tetrodes to any depth throughout the span of the experiment. Using this type of headstage gives the flexibility of optimizing the position of tetrodes for picking up the best-quality signals. (*C*) Microwire electrode array: Many microwires are arranged on a single shaft; used for recording from many single units at the same time. (*D*) Laminar microelectrode: Microelectrodes are present at varying heights on each shaft. This setup is used for recording single units from several layers of brain tissue at the same time. (*E*) Silicone-based microelectrodes: The advantage of using this type of microelectrode is the ability to integrate electronics, such as multiplexers and amplifying circuits, on the electrode system itself. (*F*) PDMS-based flexible microelectrodes: Flexible PDMS-based microelectrodes are being researched as an alternative for recording from brain areas that are otherwise inaccessible to rigid microelectrode designs. (*G*) Strip macroelectrodes: These types of macroelectrodes are placed on the cortex, most frequently in epileptic patients, for the purposes of delineating the seizure-onset zone. Electrical stimulation is also commonly performed with these electrodes to correlate physiologic function with brain area for ensuring safe resection of brain tissue in epileptic patient. Microelectrode wires can be incorporated into these (and grid) electrodes (eg, between macro contacts). (*H*) Grid macroelectrodes: These electrodes function similarly to strip macroelectrodes but have many rows of electrodes instead of one single row. (*I*) Depth macroelectrodes: These are used for recording from deeper brain structures like the hippocampus or the amygdala. Hybrid macro/micro depth electrodes of various designs are also available. (*A, B*: *Courtesy of* Dr Joseph Manns, Emory University. *E*: *From* Patterson WR, Song YK, Bull CW, et al. A microelectrode/microelectronic hybrid device for brain implantable neuroprosthesis applications. IEEE Trans Biomed Eng 2004;51(10):1845–53 [0018-9294 (Print)]; with permission. *F*: *Courtesy of* Dr Liang Guo, Georgia Institute of Technology. *G–I*: *Courtesy of* AD-Tech, Watertown, WI.)

Macroelectrodes

Macroelectrodes have dimensions on the order of a few millimeters (typically 1–5 mm), with a corresponding surface area around 1–25 mm^2, and impedance in the range of 500–1000 Ω. Consequently, they are primarily used to record LFP, ECoG, and EEG signals.

Depth macroelectrodes Depth electrodes are widely used in epileptic patients to delineate seizure foci.[22] Typical depth electrodes consist of 4 or more 1-mm contacts arranged linearly on a single shaft, separated by a distance of approximately 10 mm. In addition to recording, similar electrodes are also used for stimulation (eg, deep brain stimulation in Parkinson disease and epilepsy).[23–25] Several groups have investigated the impact of electrode geometry on recorded and stimulated volumes of brain tissue, topography, and so forth.[26,27] Recently, hybrid depth electrodes, consisting of both macroelectrodes and microwires arranged on the same shaft, have been used for simultaneous recording of LFPs and single-unit activity.[28] Image guidance techniques are used to ensure proper placement of depth electrodes.[29]

Surface macroelectrodes ECoG recordings often make use of grid and strip subdural surface electrodes.[30] In many cases subdural electrodes are used in combination with depth electrodes to delineate seizure foci. Like hybrid depth electrodes, hybrid surface electrodes — with microelectrodes interspersed between macroelectrodes — are becoming popular owing to their increased spatial resolution, and for research purposes.[31]

STIMULATION
Mechanisms of Stimulation

Little has changed in the 35 years since Ranck observed that "despite the extensive use of electrical stimulation of the central nervous system, both clinically and experimentally, there has been little concern with what cells or parts of cells are stimulated."[32] To this day, the mechanism of action of electrical stimulation on the nervous system remains poorly understood. What has become clear, however, is that many parameters of stimulation (electrode configuration, pulse width, frequency, and so forth), as well as the architectural organization of the stimulated tissue, are critical in determining its impact.

Ranck[32] noted that thresholds were lowest in myelinated axons, and progressively increased in unmyelinated axons, dendrites, and cell bodies. This point was further substantiated in a series of elegant experiments by Histed and colleagues.[33] Using simultaneous low-current 250 Hz electrical

microstimulation and 2-photon calcium imaging in mouse and cat visual cortex, the investigators were able to examine a large population of cells, free of confounding stimulus artifacts, to identify the population and location of neurons activated by cortical microstimulation. Their work revealed a sparse and distributed population of activated neurons that possessed several additional intriguing qualities. Rather than activating neurons whose cell bodies were closest to the electrode tip, cells were sparsely activated in a region surrounding the electrode, in some cases up to 4 mm away. Increasing the stimulating current amplitude increased the number of cells activated within this area, but did not activate those farther away. In fact, a large percentage of the neurons identified failed to be activated, even as their immediate neighbors were. These experiments suggest microstimulation is primarily acting on neural elements (hypothesized to be axons) as opposed to cell bodies. If axons are indeed the primary target, it is further unclear what regions are most susceptible to electrical stimulation, with the neuron initial segment[34] and nodes of Ranvier[32] being variably implicated.

Little more is known as to whether electrical stimulation primarily acts in an inhibitory or excitatory manner. One of the more accepted theories suggests that neurons adjacent to stimulating electrodes undergo long-term inactivation as a result of stimulation.[35,36] This may be based on the similarities in clinical outcome between surgical ablation and deep brain stimulation[37]; however, activation of efferent neurons, even in the context of inhibited cell bodies, has been demonstrated in several reports.[33,38,39] Indeed, even Ranck[32] noted that at high currents, elements nearby the electrode would fail to respond, whereas those in a surrounding sphere were activated. Consequently, a single stimulus could produce variable regions of activation and inhibition. The local suppression of APs and bursting activity has been noted by other groups as well: Lian and colleagues[40] found that 50-Hz sinusoidal current injected locally through a monopolar electrode could effectively block activity in a region close to the stimulation site, but was unable to completely suppress activity remotely. The mechanism underlying this suppression was posited to be through a local depolarization block from a large increase in extracellular potassium, a well-described phenomenon associated with high-frequency alternating current (AC) stimulation. Indeed, whereas electrical stimulation itself may be activating neural elements, the network effects may actually be inhibitory because of changes in electrochemical gradients, neurotransmitter depletion, or signal obfuscation.[37]

These observations have served to reinforce early indications that stimulation parameters are crucial for determining clinical outcomes. Despite this, human trials are largely based on empiric evidence and case reports.[24,37,41] Ideally, clinicians would tune treatment based on knowledge of the various interdependent properties of electrical stimulation, so as to maximize effectiveness and reduce side effects. Although there is much work to be done before the latter can become standard, current understanding should prove useful in improving clinical efficacy and research methods.

Targeting

Although gross targeting of stimuli to anatomically relevant tissue plays an important role in therapeutic outcome, local cellular cytoarchitecture has been implicated as well.[33] High-frequency deep brain stimulation (DBS) for parkinsonian tremor has primarily been targeted to neurons of the subthalamic nucleus, but it is unclear whether or not the effect is primarily mediated through the local neuron bodies or through fibers of passage.[42] Voges and colleagues[43] found the best improvements involved electrodes projecting onto fiber tracts located close to the subthalamic nucleus (STN), and recent optogenetic investigations have implicated fibers of passage to the nuclei itself.[44]

Anatomic targets may be better reflected in orthodromic and antidromic projections, as opposed to their local soma. Furthermore, orientation within these regions has the potential to be highly influential. Ranck[32] determined that more current was necessary to generate the same results if monopolar electrodes were positioned in such a way that current flow was across the axon (transverse) rather than parallel to it (longitudinal). Indeed, it was only when anodic fields were applied across the dendritic-somatic axis in slice preparations of epileptic hippocampus that seizures could be effectively suppressed.[45] Applying the field perpendicularly to this axis, however, was unable to affect activity even at high field values. Interestingly, Lian and colleagues[40] found that orientation of a monopolar electrode along the dendritic-somatic axis during AC stimulation (sinusoidal, 50 Hz, 0 direct current [DC] offset) had no effect on suppression, whereas DC stimulation was highly orientation-dependent. Higher-frequency stimulation (>50 Hz) may indeed be orientation independent,[46] despite the initial findings of Ranck.[32] This may be consequent to blockade of voltage-gated currents[47] or accumulation of extracellular potassium[41] or other biochemicals (eg,

adenosine[48]), which could occur independently from the direction of current flow.

Frequency

Frequency of stimulation, as implicated previously, can have an important influence as well. Aside from matters of orientation, different network-wide impacts have been implicated for high-frequency (roughly >50 Hz), low-frequency (<50 Hz), and DC stimulation. High-frequency stimulation can induce peripheral nerve blocks,[49] and in the subthalamic nucleus was seen to inhibit somatic neuronal activity[47] and axonal conduction in hippocampal preparations in vitro and in vivo.[50] High-frequency stimulation may thus act, in part, through a conduction blockade of pathologic activity, hence preventing spread and/or synchronization. However, effects on efferent axons independent of effects on the cell soma must be considered as well.

Low-frequency stimulation (LFS) is presumed to be excitatory in nature,[51] and was seen to reduce seizure frequency in human patients with epilepsy,[52,53] as well as in several animal models of epilepsy.[54] LFS could be inhibiting, however, as it may induce long-term depression through the alteration of synaptic weights.[53,54] It is possible that LFS activates axons, and that this activation, being asynchronous with synaptic input, generates LTD and reduces the activity of the overexcited cell. Further research is necessary to determine the exact mechanisms underlying LFS and its impact on synaptic weighting. Preliminary evidence suggests that LFS may restore normal network responses.[55]

DC electric fields can also be applied to brain tissue to suppress spontaneous epileptiform activity.[40,41,45,56] These fields are often created in vitro using parallel wires or plates. Anodic fields generate higher potentials at the cell soma vis-à-vis dendrites, resulting in positive current flow into the soma and out through the dendrites. This hyperpolarizes the soma, preventing excitation to threshold and conduction of epileptiform activity.[45] Even with the obvious difficulties with in vivo applications, there are additional drawbacks to the technique. Unbalanced charge deposition results in erosion and electrochemical tissue damage.[40] Further, suppression produces rebound excitation on removal.[45] These limitations make the application of such fields a challenge in human patients.

Polarity

Electrode configurations tend to be divided into monopolar and multipolar varieties, the most common of which is bipolar. All configurations (even so-called monopolar) consist of an anode and a cathode, with current flowing from the cathode toward the anode. In monopolar electrodes, the cathode is distant from the anode. For example, DBS stimulators will often use the pulse generator case as the anode.[24] Multipolar configurations have the anode and cathode in relative proximity, such as between neighboring contacts. Monopolar configurations thus create broader extracellular current spread than multipolar arrangements,[42] and consequently, bipolar configurations are less likely to generate unwanted side effects. Multipolar configurations allow for greater control of current distribution, enabling more precise targeting.

Waveform

Most current clinical neural stimulators make use of rectangular, charge-balanced waveforms.[57] Much of this adherence may be based on historical precedent, although charge-balancing helps reduce electrode erosion and electrochemical tissue damage.[40] Aside from potential energy savings and prolongation of stimulator battery lifetime,[57] alternative stimulus waveforms have the potential to target different regions in nervous tissue, and may be the difference between an inhibitory or an excitatory response.[50] More research must be performed to support the implications of modeling studies.[58]

Amplitude

It has long been assumed that increasing current amplitude results in a larger sphere of activated neuron bodies around the electrode contact.[32,34] However, as described earlier, stimulation results in an activation of cells in a distinct region determined by the local neuroanatomy. Higher amplitudes activate a greater number of fibers, thus increasing the number of cell bodies activated. This does *not* significantly increase the distance at which activation occurs, as it is determined by the *anatomically-defined axonal projections* of the neurons, rather than the soma's distance from the electrode tip.[33] Consequently, although higher-amplitude stimulation recruits a larger proportion of neurons, *which* neurons are influenced, and at what distance from the tip, seems to be determined by the local cytoarchitecture.

Current-Controlled Versus Voltage-Controlled Stimulation

In current-controlled stimulation, which is more commonly used experimentally,[14] current is kept constant throughout the pulse period, whereas voltage varies as a function of impedance. Lempka and colleagues[59] have shown that current-controlled stimulation may be more effective in maintaining constant voltage distribution, as the impedance of the electrode-electrolyte interface changes drastically with time. In the voltage-controlled stimulation, the voltage is kept constant while the current is allowed to vary. This method is easier to implement technically despite its lack of popularity. It is noted that some studies have shown greater efficacy of voltage-over current-controlled pulses in eliciting neural responses.[60]

ANIMAL MODELS OF EPILEPSY

Epilepsy is not one disorder, but many. Absence seizures, complex partial seizures, myotonic seizures, and so forth have varying degrees of phenomenological and electrophysiological similarities, but stem from disparate etiologies. Even within one class of seizures, generalized tonic-clonic, for instance, a single pathogenic mechanism is unlikely; rather, multiple pathogenic mechanisms beget similar seizure phenotypes.

This diversity of pathogenic mechanisms is easily illustrated by surveying the variety of animal models that generate seizures. For example, both the tetanus toxin and kainate models of epilepsy produce spontaneous generalized tonic-clonic seizures, but do so differently. Kainate, for instance, causes pathologic tissue changes in the hippocampus, similar to those found in mesial temporal sclerosis in humans,[61] and leads to frequent tonic-clonic seizures within several weeks. Tetanus toxin, after injection, likewise produces tonic-clonic seizures, but does so without a defined histologic correlate.[62–64] So, despite clear pathogenic differences, a common seizure phenotype is produced. Similar phenomenology clearly pertains to the human condition as well. This diversity of mechanisms should be kept in mind when using models to investigate the pathogenesis of epilepsy and its treatment. It is likely that seizures are the final common manifestation of several underlying pathologies. Consequently, emphasis should be placed on choosing an experimental model that closest fits each etiology, or as elegantly stated: "[T]he best material model for a cat is another, or preferably the same cat."[65]

Kindling

One of the more extensively used models of chronic temporal lobe epilepsy (TLE) is the kindling model, wherein subjects undergo daily electrical stimulation (60-Hz sine or biphasic square pulse waves at or greater than the after-discharge threshold[66]) to seizure-prone brain regions.

Kindling is a progressive phenomenon in which electrical stimulation, initially generating brief, low-frequency electrographic after-discharges without behavioral response, develop with repeated electrical stimulation over several days into long, high-frequency after-discharges with a strong convulsive response.[67–69] After many days of kindling, the subject begins to experience complex seizures with secondary generalizations. Although the progression from simple partial seizures to complex seizures is evident through stimulation in all limbic and most forebrain regions, it is most dramatic in the temporal lobe brain structure surrounding and including the amygdala.

Status Epilepticus

Status epilepticus (SE) occurs when the brain remains in a protracted state of persistent seizure, and the state can be generated electrically or chemically. The SE-induced epilepsy models have at least 3 distinct stages of development: (1) the initial status epilepticus stage lasting 6 to 12 hours, (2) The seizure-free latent period lasting a few days to several weeks, and the (3) the final and permanent stage where the animal starts having spontaneous seizures and can be considered to be epileptic.[70]

In the kainate and pilocarpine models of SE, the drug can be administered through intraperitoneal, intravenous, subcutaneous, intracerebroventricular, or intrahippocampal injections. These injections can be given either as a single large dose or as repeated smaller doses, with the latter method shown to have a lower mortality in rats.[71] The mortality rates associated with both of these models are generally very high. Although the mortality rate can be reduced by decreasing the dose of the administered drug, the chances of developing SE also decreases with reducing the drug dose. Alternatively, doses of benzodiazepine (an anticonvulsant) can be given to increase the survival rate of the animals, but this approach may also lower the chance of developing SE and subsequently having recurrent spontaneous seizures.[72]

Mazarati and colleagues[73] have shown that SE can also be induced through electrically stimulating the perforant pathway in free-running rats. This method of inducing SE had a high survival rate (90%–100%) if the stimulation durations were less than 60 minutes. Additionally, it has been shown the SE-induced epilepsy can be developed on already kindled animals either through performing 60 minutes of high-frequency stimulation of the basolateral amygdala[74,75] or through pilocarpine injections.[76]

Tetanus Toxin

Tetanus toxin is one of the oldest methods of inducing chronic experimental seizures.[77] The model involves the stereotactic injection of a minute dose of the toxin (secreted by the bacterium Clostridium tetani) into the brain. Tetanus toxin is highly toxic and hence this method needs several stringent safety controls, including vaccination of the personnel involved in the procedure and proper disposal of contaminated items. The fragile nature of the toxin also requires gentle handling, as vigorous agitations can cause the chains of the toxin to separate.

The model is highly reliable with a very low mortality rate. The rate of spontaneous seizures is very high with up to 30 seizures occurring per day for a period of 2 weeks following the first seizure.[78,79] About 90% of the rats gain remission after 6 to 8 weeks of the toxin injection. The model has also been associated with impairments in learning and memory, with these effects enduring indefinitely.[80–82]

Genetic Models

Genetic Absence Epilepsy Rats from Strasbourg (GAERS) is a genetic model of absence seizures developed by inbreeding Wistar colonies that displayed spontaneous spike-and-wave discharges. The Wistar Albino Glaxo (WAG/Rij) strain was similarly inbred in the United Kingdom and was discovered to have absence seizures.[3,83,84] The frequency of seizures in the GAERS strain is more than in the WAG/Rij rats, with the former displaying absence seizures every minute on average and the latter about 15 to 20 per hour. Both of these models have seizure characteristics that are highly reminiscent of human absence epilepsy, thus making them valuable for studying the disease in humans. Both genetic models also offer high predictability for studying the antiabsence and adverse effects of antiepileptic drugs. Studies on these models have indicated the thalamocortical circuits to be the critical generator of absence seizures.[85]

Heating/Cooling Models

The neocortical freeze lesion model in the newborn rat has been used to study the pathology of various neuronal migration disorders. This model is achieved by placing a liquid-nitrogen–cooled copper cylinder ($\sim$1 mm diameter) on the exposed calvarium of newborn rats for about 8 seconds, inducing death of immature cortical neurons and a necrotic center.[86] During the first postnatal week, newly migrating cells destined for the more superficial cortical layers invade the lesion, thus mimicking neuronal migration disorders in humans. The model has high reproducibility and low mortality rate (<5%). It is mostly used in vitro for drug screening purposes. In vivo studies are less favorable because the model does not produce spontaneous seizures.

Experimental prolonged febrile seizures in immature rats are used to study human febrile seizures. Avishai-Eliner and colleagues[87] have shown that the first year of development of the hippocampal formation in humans compares well with postnatal days 7 to 14 in rodents, making this the ideal time for eliciting febrile seizures in rats. Febrile seizures of approximately 24 minutes' duration can be elicited by maintaining hyperthermia (40–42°C) for about 30 minutes in rat pups. Like the neocortical freeze lesion model, this model too has high reproducibility and low mortality.

Alumina Gel Model

In rhesus monkeys, depending on where alumina gel is injected into the brain, 2 different types of epilepsy can be modeled. Injections into the sensorimotor cortical regions are used to model posttraumatic epilepsy, whereas injections into the temporal lobe cause complex partial seizures and neuropathological changes that mimic temporal lobe epilepsy in humans.[88]

Similar to focal motor seizures in humans, the alumina gel sensorimotor model produces spontaneous focal seizures that often become generalized. Injections made into the sensorimotor cortex are well localized, providing a good topographic focus for seizure initiation. Further, seizures begin about 4 to 8 weeks following the application of alumina gel at the sensorimotor cortex, thus giving time to analyze the neuropathological changes underlying the development of seizures.

The alumina gel model for temporal lobe epilepsy includes injections made into the hippocampus, entorhinal and perirhinal cortices, and the amygdala. Complex partial and secondary generalized seizures are observed in all cases, having marked similarities with the ictal symptoms of human temporal lobe epilepsy.

Both the sensorimotor and the temporal lobe alumina gel models suffer from high seizure variability with the subject occasionally developing status epilepticus. Further, the model is expensive, causing the number of subjects involved in any project to be low. The obvious advantage of this model is the similarity between nonhuman primates and humans.[88]

Penicillin

Penicillin has long been used as a model of simple partial seizures, because topical application to the brain's surface results in interictal spikes and epileptiform discharges. Initial use in the cat neocortex led to great insight into the neuronal basis of epilepsy, including initial observations about the paroxysmal depolarizing shift.[89] This method has been applied to several animal models, including recently the Macaca fasicularis.[90] Investigation into the mechanism underlying this effect led to the understanding that at low doses, penicillin selectively blocks GABA-mediated inhibitory postsynaptic potentials. As penicillin diffuses into a volume of only a few square millimeters, the surrounding neurons generate increased inhibitory activity in an attempt to control seizure spread. More recently, the penicillin epilepsy model has also been developed in sheep.[91]

BIDIRECTIONAL INTERFACES

Electrical stimulation is a powerful and well-studied means of influencing neural tissue, and electrical recording is one of the most prominent methods for interrogating the brain's ongoing activity. Combining these 2 modalities offers several benefits, but also presents novel challenges.

Advantages of combining stimulation and recording include the ability to better understand the effects of stimulation by monitoring the evoked activity. This information is critical to improving stimulation paradigms, as knowledge of stimulation effects are needed to rationally direct changes in stimulation parameters. This information (the neurophysiological effects of stimulation) can also be used to better understand the basic neurophysiology of epilepsy (eg, if stimulation alters the activity of a particular pathway, this information provides knowledge of how these pathways might be organized).

Another advantage of bidirectional interfaces is the direct improvement of treatment paradigms. This is best characterized by closed-loop systems, in which stimulation (the device's output) is altered by recorded neural activity (the device's input). Open-loop systems, like those conventionally used in DBS for movement disorders, use a fixed stimulation schedule that is unchanged by the brain's state. That is, whether the patient is sleeping, postprandial, or exercising, the stimulation paradigm is identical. But because of the brain's dynamism, it is easy to envision that a stimulation protocol that adapts to these changes might be more effective.

The primary challenges of bidirectional systems derive from both the physical limitations of such systems and, paradoxically, their capabilities. The main physical limitation is the problem of stimulus artifacts, described further in the following section. Briefly, trying to record an electrical signal, while simultaneously providing an extrinsic electrical signal, requires disentangling the extrinsic signal (stimulation) from the intrinsic signal (the neural activity).The other primary problem is the sheer number of possibilities unleashed by closed-loop stimulation. There are theoretically an infinite number of stimulation parameters such devices can use, and again an infinite number of control algorithms that transform recorded activity into changes in these stimulation parameters. Searching this space for the optimal parameters and algorithms remains, therefore, incredibly difficult. Guidance usually comes from existing empirical data and systems-level theorizing.

Stimulus Artifact

Recorded extracellular electrical signals are on the order of microvolts, whether single-unit APs or LFPs. Electrical stimuli, on the other hand, are typically in the range of volts, a million-fold difference in amplitude. Therefore, recording equipment designed to operate at one range seldom works well at the other. Thus, when stimulation is amplified by the recording electronics, say at $1000\times$, a 5-V pulse becomes a 5000-V input. Because this exceeds the range of the electronics, they saturate at their maximal input value, often for a duration far exceeding the stimulus pulse itself. Depending on hardware filters and the amplifier's construction, this resetting can take from milliseconds to whole seconds. During this time, the amplifier's output is not indicative of any neural signal, and therefore no useful information about the brain can be extracted.

Beyond saturation of the electronics, an additional problem is the electrical waveform produced by stimuli that are nonsaturating. This waveform is often treated as a deterministic response to stimulation (although it usually is not), and is superimposed on the intrinsic neural signals.

There are 3 primary ways experimenters are dealing with these artifacts: different hardware, specialized software, and by changing experimental design to avoid the issue entirely.

Hardware workarounds

There are many methods described for isolating and preventing stimulus artifacts from corrupting neural recordings. One of the simplest is to rely on high-resolution A/D cards and low amplification to avoid saturation. This was the approach taken by the NeuroRighter closed-loop system described by Rolston and colleagues.[2,92] Using 16-bit A/D cards and low amplification ($160\times$) reduced the amount of time amplifiers remained saturated after stimulus as compared with more complicated commercially available systems, which typically use higher gains and lower-resolution A/D cards. A further advance was attained by conducting most filtering digitally, within software. Hardware filters tend to induce ringing and store saturating charges, leading to longer stimulus artifacts. Because computers are powerful enough to conduct real-time digital filtering, analog filters are unnecessary beyond antialiasing filters. Moreover, digital filters are rapidly customizable, generally in real-time using the recording software. Additionally, storing unfiltered data allows the digital filters to be changed after the experiment, so that different analytical techniques can be used.

Because of these changes, the NeuroRighter system had artifacts lasting less than 1.0 ms, compared with 5.0 ms to 1.5 seconds for a commercial system (with the range dictated by the analog filters used).[92] Moreover, because the NeuroRighter system attained these advances by reducing the required hardware, the custom system cost one-tenth the price of an equivalent commercial system.[92]

Another method to prevent artifacts is to physically disconnect the recording electrodes from the amplifiers during the stimulus pulse, preventing the signal from reaching the amplifiers and saturating them. This disconnection usually involves a reconnection to either ground or a sample-and-hold circuit. Using high-speed switches (with switching times on the order of microseconds, far faster than the physiologic signals recorded by extracellular electrodes), the circuit will disconnect the input to the recording amplifier from the electrode and connect it to a source that stores the most recently recorded voltage (say, a few mV). When the stimulus pulse is complete, the electrode is reconnected to the recording amplifier. Using a sample-and-hold circuit rather than connecting to ground prevents an artifact induced by reconnecting the amplifier to an electrode with some DC offset, which is effectively seen by the amplifier's analog filters as another stimulus.

Software workarounds

After the data are acquired, some artifacts can be minimized digitally. These algorithms run from the simple, like template subtraction, to the complex, eg, recursive methods like Subtraction of Artifacts by Local Polynomial Approximation.[93]

Template subtraction works on the basis of recording multiple responses to a stimulation pulse.[94] These responses are then averaged to create a template for the stimulation artifact, which is then subtracted from the recorded waveform at the time of each stimulus onset. This method assumes that the stimulation artifact's waveform is static; however, hysteresis in the recording electronics and at the electrode-tissue interface can lead to changes in artifact shape over time. These changes are most acute, in our experience, at the onset of stimulation trains or when stimulating with multiple electrodes in an interlaced pattern (eg, electrode 1, then 2, then back to 1).

The dynamics of the stimulus artifact can be compensated somewhat by scaling the template to maximize its fit to the artifact to be cancelled. This approach was used by Wichmann.[95] The limitation, however, is if the waveform changes shape in addition to amplitude during experiments. In this case, scaling will be unable to adapt to artifact changes.

More complicated methods rely on curve fitting, which entails fitting an exponential or polynomial function to each detected stimulus artifact.[96] This method has the advantage of being adaptable to changes in the artifact, and is limited enough in its possible curvature that it will not cancel high-frequency components like APs. On the other hand, using a particular function (eg, exponential) assumes the artifact's shape can be completely captured by such a function. This is not always true, and poor fits lead to residual artifact.

Experimental workarounds

Experiments can also be designed so as to avoid stimulation artifacts. For instance, instead of recording activity during stimulation epochs, when artifacts interfere with the recorded signal, one could stimulate, stop stimulation, then record the stimulation's aftereffects.[97] In certain clinical situations, in fact, these aftereffects might actually be the most relevant data to analyze. Vagus nerve stimulation,[98] for example, features stimulation-free "off" times lasting several minutes, following brief "on" phases of active stimulation lasting less than a minute.

Control Algorithms

When integrating stimulation and recording into a closed-loop system, an algorithm must be chosen to translate recorded signals into the stimulator's output. For a closed-loop system to be truly closed-loop, it is necessary that stimulation affect the recorded signals. If there is no effect of stimulation, then the system is actually open-loop. Finding signals for control typically requires extracting features from the raw recorded data.

Signal features

A wide range of signal features have been used to extract seizure-related information from extracellular neural recordings. All features fall into 1 of 2 categories: discrete and continuous. Discrete features are events, like APs, interictal spikes, seizures, and other time-limited features of the signal that are either present or not (ie, binary). Continuous features are time-varying signals that can be computed for any time point of the recorded signal. Examples are signal power,[99] accumulated energy,[100] nonlinear energy,[101] entropy,[99] correlation dimension,[102] coherence,[79] and others.

Importantly, these 2 categories are not always clearly separated. On one hand, most event detection requires some sort of filtering or extraction of a time-varying signal before ultimately searching for particular events. AP detection, for example, uses high-pass filtering of the data before finding spikes,[92] and often some sort of digital referencing to reduce common-mode noise.[103] On the other hand, continuous signals can sometimes be computed from discrete events. As an example, Wagenaar and colleagues[104] used tuning based on AP firing rate to suppress epileptiform events in neural cell cultures. This firing rate is a continuous-time signal, computed by first extracting APs from the raw data.[105]

Responsive stimulation

Just as the features used for closed-loop stimulation can be of 2 kinds, discrete or continuous, so can the stimulation sequences. Responsive stimulation is the analog of the discrete, event-based features found in recordings. In responsive stimulation, stimulation sequences are triggered by the detection of a particular event. This event can be a detected seizure, as done in the NeuroPace Responsive Neurostimulation (RNS) trial, or something more abstract—the crossing of an amplitude threshold in the power spectrum, the detection of interictal spiking, changes in activity coherence, and so forth.

State control

The counterpart to responsive stimulation is state control.[106] In this method, stimulation is continuous, but altered by ongoing activity. This is in the realm of the more traditional proportional-integral-derivative-type control systems,[107] where output (stimulation, in this case) is a continuous function determined by the input (electrical recordings). Some examples of this are using firing rate to control stimulation amplitude when suppressing epileptiform bursts in culture[104] and using an adapting low-frequency electric field to suppress seizures in hippocampal slices.[56]

STIMULATION PATHWAYS AND EXAMPLES

Although optimal neural targets for electrical stimulation remain unknown, the diversity of anatomic and functional connections for separate brain structures has led to a growing array of theoretically motivated stimulation sites, ranging from subcortical nuclei to direct cortical stimulation. Subcortical nuclei are particularly attractive because of their widespread projections, offering a potential means for affecting large areas of the brain.

Limbic

The prevalence of mesial temporal lobe epilepsy is one of the prime arguments for stimulating the limbic cortex to suppress seizures. Various targets within the circuit of Papez have been tried.

Hippocampus

Several groups have conducted trials of direct stimulation of the hippocampus. Velasco and colleagues[108] studied 2 groups of patients: one with subacute (2–3 weeks) electrical stimulation of the hippocampus at 130 Hz (8 patients) and the other with chronic (3 months) stimulation (3 patients). In the subacute group, the average number of seizures declined from the time of implantation to the end of the experiment. Velasco and colleagues[108] also noted a decrease in the average number of interictal spikes. However, the investigators did not report baseline seizure and interictal spike rates, so true efficacy is unknown. Furthermore, the data are a population average, rather than examined by patient. The chronic group (3 months of hippocampal stimulation) displayed a trend toward reduced seizure counts and interictal spike rates, but without statistical significance. Overall, this small, uncontrolled trial offers provocative evidence for an effect of hippocampal stimulation, but is an insufficient basis on which to make a recommendation.

Boon and colleagues[109] also conducted an open label trial for hippocampal stimulation at 130 Hz in 10 patients. With a follow-up of 12 to 52 months, 1 patient was seizure-free, 6 patients had a reduction of greater than 50% in seizure frequency, 2 had a reduction of 30% to 49%, and 1 had no response. This was an encouraging result, which drove the case for randomized clinical trials.

Unfortunately, in the one double-blinded trial to date, using only 4 patients, there was no statistically significant effect of hippocampal DBS[110]; however, this small study did show a 15% reduction in seizure frequency. Furthermore, the stimulation frequency of 190 Hz was decidedly different from that used by Velasco and colleagues[108] and Boon and colleagues,[109] which may have led to the differential results.

Amygdala

The amygdala has major importance in models of epilepsy, as it is one of the prime targets for kindling. Kindling is the phenomenon where repeated electrical stimulation ultimately produces seizures in animal models.[66] But perhaps because of its role in kindling, direct stimulation of the amygdala has not been studied well in humans. There is a large body of evidence in animal studies, however, which suggests that low-frequency or DC stimulation might in fact suppress seizures. Weiss and colleagues[111] showed that 15-minute daily sessions of 10-μA DC stimulation of the amygdala "quenched" a rat kindling model. That is, the seizure threshold in these kindled animals increased, with the effects lasting more than 30 days after DC stimulation ended. Similar observations have been made by Goodman and colleagues[112] and Velisek and colleagues.[113]

Mammilothalamic tract and mammillary bodies

In 1984, Mirski and Ferrendelli[114] showed that sectioning of the mammillothalamic tract in guinea pigs prevented pentylenetetrazol-induced seizures from spreading. Later, Mirski and Fisher[115] showed in the rat that electrical stimulation of the mammillary bodies at 100 Hz increased seizure thresholds, ie, mammillary body stimulation made it more difficult to induce seizures in rodents. No human trials of mammillary body or mammillothalamic tract stimulation have been reported in peer-reviewed journals as of this time.

Anterior nucleus of the thalamus

The anterior nucleus of the thalamus, the target of the mammilothalamic tract and one of the inputs to the cingulate cortex, is another well-studied component of the circuit of Papez, undergoing intense investigation as a stimulation target for refractory epilepsy. It is reviewed elsewhere in this issue.

Basal Ganglia

Several groups have attempted stimulating various structures within the basal ganglia to suppress seizures, including the STN, substantia nigra pars reticulata (SNr), and caudate nucleus.

Subthalamic nucleus

Stimulation of the STN bilaterally at 130 Hz was shown to suppress the spontaneous seizures of GAERS rats (a genetic model of absence seizures) by Vercueil and colleagues[116] in the 1990s. Since then, several uncontrolled clinical trials have attempted stimulating the STN to prevent seizures in humans with modest results.[117–119] No randomized or large clinical trials have yet been reported.

Substantia nigra pars reticulata

The SNr has been a target of research for decades. Part of this attraction may stem from work by Iadarola and Gale[120] in the early 1980s. They showed that local injections of the GABA agonist muscimol into the substantia nigra prevented seizures evoked by pentylenetetrazol or bicuculline. However, these conclusions were refuted in later work by Mirski and colleagues[121] and Ono and Wada.[122]

Nevertheless, experiments show a potential role for SNr stimulation. Velisek and colleagues,[123] in particular, showed that bilateral stimulation of the SNr in young rats (postnatal day 15) suppressed flurothyl-induced clonic and tonic-clonic seizures. In adult rats, only stimulation of the anterior portion of the SNr suppressed seizures, and then only clonic, not tonic-clonic.

Caudate nucleus

Chkhenkeli[124] began experimenting with caudate stimulation in humans as early as the 1970s in Eastern Europe. In more recent work, Chkhenkeli and Chkhenkeli[125] showed that low-frequency (4–6 Hz) stimulation of the caudate reliably suppressed epileptiform activity in human subjects. Studies in the alumina gel nonhuman primate model of epilepsy also showed ameliorative effects of stimulation, although at the higher frequency of 100 Hz rather than Chkhenkeli's 4 to 6 Hz.

Cerebellum

Stimulation of the cerebellum to suppress seizures has been attempted in humans since the 1970s, when Irving S. Cooper and colleagues reported their experience.[126–129] However, their data and conclusions were frequently called into question by other researchers, particularly in double-blind trials.[130–132] Cooper recounts these refutations with chagrin in his memoirs.[133] Most recently, a small double-blind trial was conducted in Mexico by Velasco and colleagues.[134] In this study, 10-Hz stimulation of the cerebellum reduced seizures by 33% in 3 patients with generalized tonic-clonic seizures.

Locus Coeruleus

Stimulation of the locus coeruleus (LC), the principal site of production of norepinephrine in the brainstem, was attempted in the 1970s by Feinstein and colleagues.[135] They implanted 2 patients with epilepsy and 1 with cerebral palsy and measured levels of 3-methoxy-4-hydroxyphenylethyleneglycol to verify that the activation of the LC. Although a notable reduction in spasticity was achieved, the reduction in seizures was not robust enough to be supported statistically.[135]

SUMMARY

A common set of issues surrounds every attempt to use electrical stimulation to treat epilepsy. What type of electrodes should be used? Where should they be located? What stimulation parameters will be most effective? Which groups of patients will most likely benefit?

Currently, these questions have no definitive answers, but it is our hope that continued research will ultimately provide us the tools to offer rational therapy to our patients. Extracellular recordings will continue to provide insight into the mechanism of stimulation, bidirectional interfaces will offer new means of interacting with nervous tissue in complex and nuanced ways, and animal models will continue illuminating which modes of manipulating the brain are most promising for future experiments in humans.

ACKNOWLEDGMENTS

This work was funded by the Wallace H. Coulter Foundation, the Epilepsy Research Foundation, a Neurology/Biomedical Engineering seed grant from Emory University and Georgia Tech, a University Research Council grant from Emory University, the National Institute of General Medical Sciences (NIGMS) for J.D.R. and N.G.L (gs1). (GM08169), and from the National Institute of Neurologic Disorders and Stroke (NINDS), a Ruth L. Kirschstein National Research Service Award to J.D.R (gs2). (NS060392), a translational research fellowship to J.D.R (gs3). (NS007480), a career development award to R.E.G (gs4). (NS046322), and a research grant to R.E.G. (NS054809). The funders had no role in study design, data collection and analysis, decision to publish, or preparation of the manuscript.

REFERENCES

1. Lockman J, Fisher RS. Therapeutic brain stimulation for epilepsy. Neurol Clin 2009;27(4):1031–40.
2. Rolston JD, Gross RE, Potter SM. Closed-loop, open-source electrophysiology. Front Neurosci 2010;4:31.
3. Amirnovin R, Williams ZM, Cosgrove GR, et al. Experience with microelectrode guided subthalamic nucleus deep brain stimulation. Neurosurgery 2006; 58(Suppl 1):ONS96–102 [discussion: ONS96–102].

4. Cogan SF. Neural stimulation and recording electrodes. Annu Rev Biomed Eng 2008;10:275–309.

5. Desai SA, Rolston JD, Guo L, et al. Improving impedance of implantable microwire multielectrode arrays by ultrasonic electroplating of durable platinum black. Front Neuroeng 2010;3:5.

6. Lewicki MS. A review of methods for spike sorting: the detection and classification of neural action potentials. Network 1998;9(4):R53–78.

7. Stark E, Abeles M. Predicting movement from multiunit activity. J Neurosci 2007;27(31):8387–94.

8. Katzner S, Nauhaus I, Benucci A, et al. Local origin of field potentials in visual cortex. Neuron 2009; 61(1):35–41.

9. Berens P, Keliris GA, Ecker AS, et al. Comparing the feature selectivity of the gamma-band of the local field potential and the underlying spiking activity in primate visual cortex. Front Syst Neurosci 2008;2:2.

10. Kreiman G, Hung CP, Kraskov A, et al. Object selectivity of local field potentials and spikes in the macaque inferior temporal cortex. Neuron 2006;49(3):433–45.

11. Liu J, Newsome WT. Local field potential in cortical area MT: stimulus tuning and behavioral correlations. J Neurosci 2006;26(30):7779–90.

12. Leuthardt EC, Schalk G, Wolpaw JR, et al. A brain-computer interface using electrocorticographic signals in humans. J Neural Eng 2004; 1(2):63–71.

13. Smith SJ. EEG in the diagnosis, classification, and management of patients with epilepsy. J Neurol Neurosurg Psychiatry 2005;76(Suppl 2):ii2–7.

14. Merrill DR, Bikson M, Jefferys JG. Electrical stimulation of excitable tissue: design of efficacious and safe protocols. J Neurosci Methods 2005;141(2): 171–98.

15. Loeb GE, Peck RA, Martyniuk J. Toward the ultimate metal microelectrode. J Neurosci Methods 1995;63(1–2):175–83.

16. Gray CM, Maldonado PE, Wilson M, et al. Tetrodes markedly improve the reliability and yield of multiple single-unit isolation from multi-unit recordings in cat striate cortex. J Neurosci Methods 1995; 63(1–2):43–54.

17. Bartels J, Andreasen D, Ehirim P, et al. Neurotrophic electrode: method of assembly and implantation into human motor speech cortex. J Neurosci Methods 2008;174(2):168–76.

18. Hoogerwerf AC, Wise KD. A three-dimensional microelectrode array for chronic neural recording. IEEE Trans Biomed Eng 1994;41(12): 1136–46.

19. Patterson WR, Song YK, Bull CW, et al. A microelectrode/microelectronic hybrid device for brain implantable neuroprosthesis applications. IEEE Trans Biomed Eng 2004;51(10):1845–53.

20. Guo L, DeWeerth SP. High-density stretchable electronics: toward an integrated multilayer composite. Adv Mater 2010;22(36):4030–3.

21. Guo L, Deweerth SP. PDMS-based conformable microelectrode arrays with selectable novel 3-D microelectrode geometries for surface stimulation and recording. Conf Proc IEEE Eng Med Biol Soc 2009;2009:1623–6.

22. Behrens E, Zentner J, van Roost D, et al. Subdural and depth electrodes in the presurgical evaluation of epilepsy. Acta Neurochir (Wien) 1994;128(1–4): 84–7.

23. Bronstein JM, Tagliati M, Alterman RL, et al. Deep brain stimulation for Parkinson disease: an expert consensus and review of key issues. Arch Neurol 2011;68(2):165.

24. Fisher R, Salanova V, Witt T, et al. Electrical stimulation of the anterior nucleus of thalamus for treatment of refractory epilepsy. Epilepsia 2010;51(5): 899–908.

25. Sun FT, Morrell MJ, Wharen RE Jr, et al. Responsive cortical stimulation for the treatment of epilepsy. Neurotherapeutics 2008;5(1):68–74.

26. Butson CR, Cooper SE, Henderson JM, et al. Patient-specific analysis of the volume of tissue activated during deep brain stimulation. Neuroimage 2007;34(2):661–70.

27. Grill WM, Wei XF. High efficiency electrodes for deep brain stimulation. Conf Proc IEEE Eng Med Biol Soc 2009;2009:3298–301.

28. Worrell GA, Gardner AB, Stead SM, et al. High-frequency oscillations in human temporal lobe: simultaneous microwire and clinical macroelectrode recordings. Brain 2008;131(Pt 4):928–37.

29. Yeh HS, Taha JM, Tobler WD. Implantation of intracerebral depth electrodes for monitoring seizures using the Pelorus stereotactic system guided by magnetic resonance imaging. Technical note. J Neurosurg 1993;78(1):138–41.

30. Wyler AR, Ojemann GA, Lettich E, et al. Subdural strip electrodes for localizing epileptogenic foci. J Neurosurg 1984;60(6):1195–200.

31. Van Gompel JJ, Stead SM, Giannini C, et al. Phase I trial: safety and feasibility of intracranial electroencephalography using hybrid subdural electrodes containing macro- and microelectrode arrays. Neurosurg Focus 2008;25(3):E23.

32. Ranck JB Jr. Which elements are excited in electrical stimulation of mammalian central nervous system: a review. Brain Res 1975;98(3):417–40.

33. Histed MH, Bonin V, Reid RC. Direct activation of sparse, distributed populations of cortical neurons by electrical microstimulation. Neuron 2009;63(4): 508–22.

34. Tehovnik EJ. Electrical stimulation of neural tissue to evoke behavioral responses. J Neurosci Methods 1996;65(1):1–17.

35. Boon P, Raedt R, de Herdt V, et al. Electrical stimulation for the treatment of epilepsy. Neurotherapeutics 2009;6(2):218–27.

36. Skarpaas TL, Morrell MJ. Intracranial stimulation therapy for epilepsy. Neurotherapeutics 2009;6(2): 238–43.

37. Benabid AL. What the future holds for deep brain stimulation. Expert Rev Med Devices 2007;4(6): 895–903.

38. Miocinovic S, Parent M, Butson CR, et al. Computational analysis of subthalamic nucleus and lenticular fasciculus activation during therapeutic deep brain stimulation. J Neurophysiol 2006;96(3): 1569–80.

39. Lafreniere-Roula M, Hutchison WD, Lozano AM, et al. Microstimulation-induced inhibition as a tool to aid targeting the ventral border of the subthalamic nucleus. J Neurosurg 2009;111(4):724–8.

40. Lian J, Bikson M, Sciortino C, et al. Local suppression of epileptiform activity by electrical stimulation in rat hippocampus in vitro. J Physiol 2003;547(2): 427–34.

41. Sunderam S, Gluckman B, Reato D, et al. Toward rational design of electrical stimulation strategies for epilepsy control. Epilepsy Behav 2010;17(1): 6–22.

42. Kuncel AM, Grill WM. Selection of stimulus parameters for deep brain stimulation. Clin Neurophysiol 2004;115(11):2431–41.

43. Voges J, Volkmann J, Allert N, et al. Bilateral high-frequency stimulation in the subthalamic nucleus for the treatment of Parkinson disease: correlation of therapeutic effect with anatomical electrode position. J Neurosurg 2002;96(2):269–79.

44. Gradinaru V, Mogri M, Thompson KR, et al. Optical deconstruction of parkinsonian neural circuitry. Science 2009;324(5925):354–9.

45. Ghai RS, Bikson M, Durand DM. Effects of applied electric fields on low-calcium epileptiform activity in the CA1 region of rat hippocampal slices. J Neurophysiol 2000;84(1):274–80.

46. Bikson M, Lian J, Hahn PJ, et al. Suppression of epileptiform activity by high frequency sinusoidal fields in rat hippocampal slices. J Physiol 2001; 531(1):181–91.

47. Beurrier C, Bioulac B, Audin J, et al. High-frequency stimulation produces a transient blockade of voltage-gated currents in subthalamic neurons. J Neurophysiol 2001;85(4):1351–6.

48. Zhong XL, Yu JT, Zhang Q, et al. Deep brain stimulation for epilepsy in clinical practice and in animal models. Brain Res Bull 2011;85(3–4): 81–8.

49. Gerges M, Foldes EL, Ackermann DM, et al. Frequency- and amplitude-transitioned waveforms mitigate the onset response in high-frequency nerve block. J Neural Eng 2010;7(6):066003.

50. Jensen AL, Durand DM. High frequency stimulation can block axonal conduction. Exp Neurol 2009; 220(1):57–70.

51. Theodore WH, Fisher RS. Brain stimulation for epilepsy. Lancet Neurol 2004;3(2):111–8.

52. Durand DM. Control of seizure activity by electrical stimulation: effect of frequency. Conf Proc IEEE Eng Med Biol Soc 2009;2009:2375.

53. Schrader LM, Stern JM, Wilson CL, et al. Low frequency electrical stimulation through subdural electrodes in a case of refractory status epilepticus. Clin Neurophysiol 2006;117(4):781–8.

54. Kile KB, Tian N, Durand DM. Low frequency stimulation decreases seizure activity in a mutation model of epilepsy. Epilepsia 2010;51(9):1745–53.

55. Andrews RJ. Neuromodulation. Ann N Y Acad Sci 2010;1199(1):204–11.

56. Gluckman BJ, Nguyen H, Weinstein SL, et al. Adaptive electric field control of epileptic seizures. J Neurosci 2001;21(2):590–600.

57. Foutz TJ, McIntyre CC. Evaluation of novel stimulus waveforms for deep brain stimulation. J Neural Eng 2010;7(6):066008.

58. McIntyre CC, Grill WM. Extracellular stimulation of central neurons: influence of stimulus waveform and frequency on neuronal output. J Neurophysiol 2002;88(4):1592–604.

59. Lempka SF, Miocinovic S, Johnson MD, et al. In vivo impedance spectroscopy of deep brain stimulation electrodes. J Neural Eng 2009;6(4): 46001.

60. Wagenaar DA, Pine J, Potter SM. Effective parameters for stimulation of dissociated cultures using multi-electrode arrays. J Neurosci Methods 2004; 138(1–2):27–37.

61. Ben-Ari Y. Limbic seizure and brain damage produced by kainic acid: mechanisms and relevance to human temporal lobe epilepsy. Neuroscience 1985;14(2):375–403.

62. Mellanby J, George G, Robinson A, et al. Epileptiform syndrome in rats produced by injecting tetanus toxin into the hippocampus. J Neurol Neurosurg Psychiatry 1977;40(4):404–14.

63. Jefferys JG, Evans BJ, Hughes SA, et al. Neuropathology of the chronic epileptic syndrome induced by intrahippocampal tetanus toxin in rat: preservation of pyramidal cells and incidence of dark cells. Neuropathol Appl Neurobiol 1992; 18(1):53–70.

64. Benke TA, Swann J. The tetanus toxin model of chronic epilepsy. Adv Exp Med Biol 2004;548: 226–38.

65. Rosenbluth A, Weiner N. The role of models in science. Philos Sci 1945;12:316–21.

66. Pitkanen A, Schwartzkroin PA, Moshé SL. Models of seizures and epilepsy. Burlington (MA): Elsevier Academic Press; 2006.

67. Goddard GV, McIntyre DC, Leech CK. A permanent change in brain function resulting from daily electrical stimulation. Exp Neurol 1969;25(3):295–330.

68. McIntyre DC. Differential amnestic effect of cortical vs. amygdaloid elicited convulsions in rats. Physiol Behav 1970;5(7):747–53.

69. McIntyre DC, Saari M, Pappas BA. Potentiation of amygdala kindling in adult or infants rats by injections of 6-hydroxydopamine. Exp Neurol 1979; 63(3):527–44.

70. Dudek FE, Hellier JL, Williams PA, et al. The course of cellular alterations associated with the development of spontaneous seizures after status epilepticus. Prog Brain Res 2002;135:53–65.

71. Hellier JL, Patrylo PR, Buckmaster PS, et al. Recurrent spontaneous motor seizures after repeated low-dose systemic treatment with kainate: assessment of a rat model of temporal lobe epilepsy. Epilepsy Res 1998;31(1):73–84.

72. Lemos T, Cavalheiro EA. Suppression of pilocarpine-induced status epilepticus and the late development of epilepsy in rats. Exp Brain Res 1995; 102(3):423–8.

73. Mazarati AM, Wasterlain CG, Sankar R, et al. Self-sustaining status epilepticus after brief electrical stimulation of the perforant path. Brain Res 1998; 801(1–2):251–3.

74. McIntyre DC, Nathanson D, Edson N. A new model of partial status epilepticus based on kindling. Brain Res 1982;250(1):53–63.

75. McIntyre DC, Stokes KA, Edson N. Status epilepticus following stimulation of a kindled hippocampal focus in intact and commissurotomized rats. Exp Neurol 1986;94(3):554–70.

76. Buterbaugh GG, Michelson HB, Keyser DO. Status epilepticus facilitated by pilocarpine in amygdala-kindled rats. Exp Neurol 1986;94(1):91–102.

77. Roux E, Borrel A. Tétanos cérébral et immunité contre le tétanos. Ann Inst Pasteur 1898;4: 225–39.

78. Jefferys JG, Borck C, Mellanby J. Chronic focal epilepsy induced by intracerebral tetanus toxin. Ital J Neurol Sci 1995;16(1–2):27–32.

79. Rolston JD, Laxpati NG, Gutekunst CA, et al. Spontaneous and evoked high-frequency oscillations in the tetanus toxin model of epilepsy. Epilepsia 2010; 51(11):2289–96.

80. George G, Mellanby J. Memory deficits in an experimental hippocampal epileptiform syndrome in rats. Exp Neurol 1982;75(3):678–89.

81. Jefferys JG, Williams SF. Physiological and behavioural consequences of seizures induced in the rat by intrahippocampal tetanus toxin. Brain 1987; 110(Pt 2):517–32.

82. Mellanby J, Oliva M, Peniket A, et al. The effect of experimental epilepsy induced by injection of tetanus toxin into the amygdala of the rat on eating behaviour and response to novelty. Behav Brain Res 1999;100(1–2):113–22.

83. van Luijtelaar EL, Coenen AM. Two types of electrocortical paroxysms in an inbred strain of rats. Neurosci Lett 1986;70(3):393–7.

84. Vergnes M, Marescaux C, Micheletti G, et al. Spontaneous paroxysmal electroclinical patterns in rat: a model of generalized non-convulsive epilepsy. Neurosci Lett 1982;33(1):97–101.

85. Danober L, Deransart C, Depaulis A, et al. Pathophysiological mechanisms of genetic absence epilepsy in the rat. Prog Neurobiol 1998;55(1): 27–57.

86. Dvořák K, Feit J, Juránková Z. Experimentally induced focal microgyria and status verrucosus deformis in rats—Pathogenesis and interrelation histological and autoradiographical study. Acta Neuropathol 1978;44(2):121–9.

87. Avishai-Eliner S, Brunson KL, Sandman CA, et al. Stressed-out, or in (utero)? Trends Neurosci 2002; 25(10):518–24.

88. Ribak CE, Seress L, Weber P, et al. Alumina gel injections into the temporal lobe of rhesus monkeys cause complex partial seizures and morphological changes found in human temporal lobe epilepsy. J Comp Neurol 1998;401(2):266–90.

89. Fisher RS. Animal models of the epilepsies. Brain Res Rev 1989;14(3):245–78.

90. Blauwblomme T, Piallat B, Fourcade A, et al. Cortical stimulation of the epileptogenic zone for the treatment of focal motor seizures: an experimental study in the non human primate. Neurosurgery 2011;68(2):482–90.

91. Stypulkowski PH, Giftakis JE, Billstrom TM. Development of a large animal model for investigation of deep brain stimulation for epilepsy. Stereotact Funct Neurosurg 2011;89(2):111–22.

92. Rolston JD, Gross RE, Potter SM. A low-cost multielectrode system for data acquisition enabling real-time closed-loop processing with rapid recovery from stimulation artifacts. Front Neuroeng 2009;2:12.

93. Wagenaar DA, Potter SM. Real-time multi-channel stimulus artifact suppression by local curve fitting. J Neurosci Methods 2002;120(2):113–20.

94. Hashimoto T, Elder CM, Vitek JL. A template subtraction method for stimulus artifact removal in high-frequency deep brain stimulation. J Neurosci Methods 2002;113(2):181–6.

95. Wichmann T. A digital averaging method for removal of stimulus artifacts in neurophysiologic experiments. J Neurosci Methods 2000;98(1):57–62.

96. Erez Y, Tischler H, Moran A, et al. Generalized framework for stimulus artifact removal. J Neurosci Methods 2010;191(1):45–59.

97. Benazzouz A, Piallat B, Pollak P, et al. Responses of substantia nigra pars reticulata and globus pallidus complex to high frequency stimulation of the

subthalamic nucleus in rats: electrophysiological data. Neurosci Lett 1995;189(2):77–80.

98. Navas M, Navarrete EG, Pascual JM, et al. Treatment of refractory epilepsy in adult patients with right-sided vagus nerve stimulation. Epilepsy Res 2010;90(1–2):1–7.

99. Greene BR, Faul S, Marnane WP, et al. A comparison of quantitative EEG features for neonatal seizure detection. Clin Neurophysiol 2008;119(6):1248–61.

100. Guo L, Rivero D, Dorado J, et al. Automatic epileptic seizure detection in EEGs based on line length feature and artificial neural networks. J Neurosci Methods 2010;191(1):101–9.

101. D'Alessandro M, Esteller R, Vachtsevanos G, et al. Epileptic seizure prediction using hybrid feature selection over multiple intracranial EEG electrode contacts: a report of four patients. IEEE Trans Biomed Eng 2003;50(5):603–15.

102. Elger CE, Lehnertz K. Seizure prediction by nonlinear time series analysis of brain electrical activity. Eur J Neurosci 1998;10(2):786–9.

103. Rolston JD, Gross RE, Potter SM. Common median referencing for improved action potential detection with multielectrode arrays. In: 31st Annual International Conference of the IEEE Engineering in Medicine and Biology Society. Minneapolis (MN), September 3–6, 2009.

104. Wagenaar DA, et al. Controlling bursting in cortical cultures with closed-loop multi-electrode stimulation. J Neurosci 2005;25(3):680–8.

105. Dayan P, Abbott LF. Theoretical neuroscience: computational and mathematical modeling of neural systems. Computational neuroscience. Cambridge (MA): Massachusetts Institute of Technology Press; 2001. xv. p. 460.

106. Schachter SC, Guttag J, Schiff SJ, et al; Summit Contributors. Advances in the application of technology to epilepsy: the CIMIT/NIO Epilepsy Innovation Summit. Epilepsy Behav 2009;16(1):3–46.

107. Åström KJ, Murray RM. Feedback systems: an introduction for scientists and engineers. Princeton (NJ): Princeton University Press; 2008. xii. p. 396.

108. Velasco AL, Velasco M, Velasco F, et al. Subacute and chronic electrical stimulation of the hippocampus on intractable temporal lobe seizures: preliminary report. Arch Med Res 2000;31(3):316–28.

109. Boon P, Vonck K, De Herdt V, et al. Deep brain stimulation in patients with refractory temporal lobe epilepsy. Epilepsia 2007;48(8):1551–60.

110. Tellez-Zenteno JF, McLachlan RS, Parrent A, et al. Hippocampal electrical stimulation in mesial temporal lobe epilepsy. Neurology 2006;66(10):1490–4.

111. Weiss SR, Eidsath A, Li XL, et al. Quenching revisited: low level direct current inhibits amygdala-kindled seizures. Exp Neurol 1998;154(1):185–92.

112. Goodman JH, Berger RE, Tcheng TK. Preemptive low-frequency stimulation decreases the incidence of amygdala-kindled seizures. Epilepsia 2005;46(1):1–7.

113. Velisek L, Veliskova J, Stanton PK. Low-frequency stimulation of the kindling focus delays basolateral amygdala kindling in immature rats. Neurosci Lett 2002;326(1):61–3.

114. Mirski MA, Ferrendelli JA. Interruption of the mammillothalamic tract prevents seizures in guinea pigs. Science 1984;226(4670):72–4.

115. Mirski MA, Fisher RS. Electrical stimulation of the mammillary nuclei increases seizure threshold to pentylenetetrazol in rats. Epilepsia 1994;35(6):1309–16.

116. Vercueil L, Benazzouz A, Deransart C, et al. High-frequency stimulation of the sub-thalamic nucleus suppresses absence seizures in the rat: comparison with neurotoxic lesions. Epilepsy Res 1998;31(1):39–46.

117. Lee KJ, Jang KS, Shon YM. Chronic deep brain stimulation of subthalamic and anterior thalamic nuclei for controlling refractory partial epilepsy. Acta Neurochir Suppl 2006;99:87–91.

118. Handforth A, DeSalles AA, Krahl SE. Deep brain stimulation of the subthalamic nucleus as adjunct treatment for refractory epilepsy. Epilepsia 2006;47:1239–41.

119. Benabid AL, Minotti L, Koudsié A, et al. Antiepileptic effect of high-frequency stimulation of the subthalamic nucleus (corpus luysi) in a case of medically intractable epilepsy caused by focal dysplasia: a 30-month follow-up: technical case report. Neurosurgery 2002;50(6):1385–91 [discussion: 1391–2].

120. Iadarola MJ, Gale K. Substantia nigra: site of anticonvulsant activity mediated by gamma-aminobutyric acid. Science 1982;218(4578):1237–40.

121. Mirski MA, McKeon AC, Ferrendelli JA. Anterior thalamus and substantia nigra: two distinct structures mediating experimental generalized seizures. Brain Res 1986;397(2):377–80.

122. Ono K, Wada JA. Facilitation of premotor cortical seizure development by intranigral muscimol. Brain Res 1987;405(1):183–6.

123. Velisek L, Veliskova J, Moshe SL. Electrical stimulation of substantia nigra pars reticulata is anticonvulsant in adult and young male rats. Exp Neurol 2002;173(1):145–52.

124. Chkhenkeli SA. The inhibitory influence of the nucleus caudatus electrostimulation on the human's amygdalar and hippocampal activity at temporal lobe epilepsy. Bull Ga Acad Sci 1978;4/6:406–11.

125. Chkhenkeli SA, Chkhenkeli IS. Effects of therapeutic stimulation of nucleus caudatus on epileptic electrical activity of brain in patients with intractable epilepsy. Stereotact Funct Neurosurg 1997;69(1–4 Pt 2):221–4.

126. Cooper IS, Amin I, Gilman S. The effect of chronic cerebellar stimulation upon epilepsy in man. Trans Am Neurol Assoc 1973;98:192–6.

127. Cooper IS, Amin I, Riklan M, et al. Chronic cerebellar stimulation in epilepsy. Clinical and anatomical studies. Arch Neurol 1976;33(8):559–70.

128. Cooper IS, Amin I, Upton A, et al. Safety and efficacy of chronic stimulation. Neurosurgery 1977; 1(2):203–5.

129. Cooper IS, Upton AR. Effects of cerebellar stimulation on epilepsy, the EEG and cerebral palsy in man. Electroencephalogr Clin Neurophysiol Suppl 1978;34:349–54.

130. Van Buren JM, Wood JH, Oakley J, et al. Preliminary evaluation of cerebellar stimulation by double-blind stimulation and biological criteria in the treatment of epilepsy. J Neurosurg 1978;48(3):407–16.

131. Wright GD, McLellan DL, Brice JG. A double-blind trial of chronic cerebellar stimulation in twelve patients with severe epilepsy. J Neurol Neurosurg Psychiatry 1984;47(8):769–74.

132. Krauss GL, Fisher RS. Cerebellar and thalamic stimulation for epilepsy. Adv Neurol 1993;63:231–45.

133. Cooper IS. The vital probe: my life as a brain surgeon. 1st edition. New York: Norton; 1981. p. 346.

134. Velasco F, Carrillo-Ruiz JD, Brito F, et al. Double-blind, randomized controlled pilot study of bilateral cerebellar stimulation for treatment of intractable motor seizures. Epilepsia 2005;46(7): 1071–81.

135. Feinstein B, Gleason CA, Libet B. Stimulation of locus coeruleus in man. Preliminary trials for spasticity and epilepsy. Stereotact Funct Neurosurg 1989;52(1):26–41.

Efficacy of Vagus Nerve Stimulation for Epilepsy by Patient Age, Epilepsy Duration, and Seizure Type

Dario J. Englot, MD, PhD, Edward F. Chang, MD,
Kurtis I. Auguste, MD*

KEYWORDS

• Epilepsy • Outcomes • Seizures • Surgery
• Vagus nerve stimulation

Nearly 1% of the population has epilepsy, and approximately 30% of these patients are refractory to medical therapy, resulting in significant morbidity.[1] Although resection of an epileptic focus can be curative in selected patients with intractable epilepsy, others are poor surgical candidates because of multifocal seizure origin or eloquence near epileptic foci.[2] In 1997, the US Food and Drug Administration (FDA) approved left-sided vagus nerve stimulation (VNS) as an adjunctive treatment of medically refractory partial epilepsy, and stimulators have now been implanted in more than 60,000 patients.[3–5] The neurobiological mechanisms of VNS in epilepsy remain poorly understood, although data from humans and animals have suggested that vagal stimulation may desynchronize activity and decrease abnormal spiking patterns on electroencephalography.[6–8] Two randomized controlled trials have evaluated the efficacy of VNS in epilepsy, finding a reduction in seizure frequency of between 23% and 57% after 3 months of therapy.[9,10] However, controversy regarding the utility of VNS in epilepsy persists because of inconsistent results, small sample sizes, and short duration of follow-up in many clinical studies. In particular, although VNS was approved in the United States only for patients aged 12 years and more with partial seizures, its benefit in children and patients with generalized epilepsy syndromes remains unclear. Furthermore, it is not known whether preoperative duration of epilepsy or seizure semiology predicts varied clinical response to VNS therapy.

In this article, we provide a retrospective analysis of seizure outcomes after VNS for pharmacologically resistant epilepsy from a large patient registry. Clinical response to VNS was evaluated at various time points after device implantation, and patient age, duration of epilepsy, predominant seizure type, and the presence of epileptic encephalopathy were investigated as potential prognostic indicators of a favorable outcome.

MATERIALS AND METHODS
Patient Outcome Registry Data Collection

All data were obtained from the VNS therapy patient outcome registry maintained by the manufacturer of the device, Cyberonics, Inc (Houston, TX, USA). This database was established in 1999, after FDA approval of VNS for epilepsy in 1997, to systematically monitor patient outcomes. Data were voluntarily provided by 1285 prescribing physicians from 978 centers (911 in the United

The authors have no conflicts of interest to disclose.
Department of Neurological Surgery, Epilepsy Center, University of California, San Francisco, CA, USA
* Corresponding author. Department of Neurological Surgery, University of California, San Francisco, 505 Parnassus Avenue, Box 0112, San Francisco, CA 94143-0112.
E-mail address: augustek@neurosurg.ucsf.edu

States and Canada and 67 international) at patients' preoperative baseline and at various intervals during therapy. Previous investigators have authenticated the integrity of the systems for collecting and processing registry data using an independent auditing agency.[11] The database was queried in March 2011 for all seizure outcomes reported at 3, 6, 12, and 24 months after VNS device implantation compared with preoperative baseline. Overall decrease in seizure frequency and response rates to VNS therapy were measured at each follow-up, with favorable clinical response defined as a decrease in seizure frequency of 50% or more versus baseline. Outcomes were stratified by (1) age (<6, 6–18, or >18 years), (2) preoperative duration of epilepsy (<5, 5–10, or >10 years), (3) predominant preoperative seizure type (aura-only, simple-partial, complex-partial, primary generalized tonic-clonic, secondarily generalized tonic-clonic, atonic, absence, other, or multiple predominant seizure types), and (4) the presence or absence of Lennox-Gastaut syndrome or other epileptic encephalopathy.

Statistical Analysis

Between-group comparisons for seizure outcomes after 1 year of VNS therapy were performed across subgroups of patients using Pearson chi-square test. Variables found to be significant on chi-square test were then further interrogated using binary logistic regression to elucidate possible predictors of seizure outcome. Odds ratios (ORs) were calculated with a 95% confidence interval (CI). The level of significance was set at 0.05 for all analyses. Statistical analysis was performed using SPSS version 17 (IBM Corp, Armonk, NY, USA).

RESULTS

Seizure outcomes were identified and analyzed across 4483, 3040, 2698, and 1104 patients at 3, 6, 12, and 24 months after VNS therapy, respectively. Outcomes for all patients are summarized in **Table 1**. Three months after initiation of VNS therapy, patients experienced a median decrease of 46% in seizure frequency compared with baseline, and 1990 of 4483 patients (44%) responded favorably to therapy by achieving a decrease of 50% or more in seizures (see **Table 1**). At 1- and 2-year follow-up, individuals experienced 56% and 62% fewer seizures (median), respectively, with 53% and 56% of patients achieving notable benefit from therapy, respectively (see **Table 1**). These results suggest that the clinical benefit of VNS for epilepsy progressively increases with treatment duration, with slightly greater than half of all patients responding to VNS after 1 year of therapy.

We next analyzed whether or not age predicted response to VNS, as summarized in **Fig. 1**. After 1 year of therapy, children younger than 6 years and of 6 to 18 years experienced 60% fewer seizures (median) compared with baseline, whereas adults (>18 years old) achieved a decrease of 53% in seizure frequency (see **Fig. 1**A). Rates of clinical response ($\geq$seizure reduction) differed significantly across the 3 age groups ($\chi^2 = 8.1$, $P = .018$, 1-year follow-up). Specifically, 56% to 57% of children but only 51% of adults responded favorably to VNS at 1 year of treatment (see **Fig. 1**B). Overall, age of 18 years or less significantly predicted a higher likelihood of favorable response with an OR of 1.27 (95% CI, 1.07–1.50; $P = .006$). These findings suggest that despite the initial FDA approval of VNS for adults and adolescents, children may receive the greatest clinical benefit from therapy.

We next investigated the duration of epilepsy before VNS device implantation as a potential predictor of clinical response to VNS. Outcomes were stratified across individuals with less than 5, 5 to 10, and more than 10 years of preoperative seizures (**Fig. 2**). We noted that individuals with a shorter duration of epilepsy tended to respond more favorably to VNS, experiencing a larger decrease in seizures after 1 to 2 years of therapy compared with those with longer seizure histories

Table 1
Overall response to VNS implantation

Duration of Implant (mo)	N	Median % Decrease in Seizure Frequency (Interquartile Range)	Number of Responders (%)[a]
3	4483	46 (77)	1990 (44)
6	3040	50 (82)	1498 (49)
12	2698	56 (76)	1432 (53)
24	1104	62 (72)	619 (56)

[a] Defined by a decrease of 50% or more in seizure frequency versus baseline.

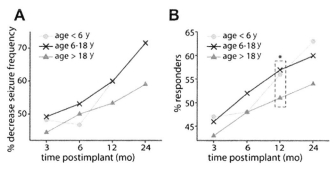

Fig. 1. Pediatric patients achieve better response to VNS than adults. (*A*) Median percentage decrease in seizure frequency at 3, 6, 12, and 24 months after VNS implantation compared with preoperative baseline, stratified by age in years. (*B*) Percentage of patients who clinically responded to VNS, achieving a decrease of 50% or more in seizure frequency after VNS compared with baseline. After 1 year of therapy, children (age<18 years) experienced a significantly higher rate of response (P<.05) than adults (*asterisk*). N at 3, 6, 12, and 24 months are 238, 155, 111, and 30 for age less than 6 years; 1422, 937, 831, and 294 for age 6 to 18 years; and 2823, 1948, 1756, and 780 for age more than 18 years, respectively.

(see **Fig. 2**A). Also, responder rates at 1 year (see **Fig. 2**B) differed significantly by epilepsy duration ($\chi^2 = 6.7$, $P = .035$). Overall, a seizure history of 10 years or less predicted a somewhat higher likelihood of favorable clinical response (56%) than a history of more than 10 years of epilepsy (52%) (OR, 1.19; 95% CI, 1.00–1.41). This difference approached, but did not reach, statistical significance ($P = .053$). Thus, although clinical effects of VNS are relatively similar between individuals with a shorter or longer epilepsy history, additional benefit may be gained from early intervention.

Next, given the initial FDA approval of VNS for patients with partial epilepsy only, we examined seizure outcomes after therapy stratified by predominant preoperative seizure type. As shown in **Fig. 3**, rates of clinical response differed significantly across various seizure types ($\chi^2 = 40.0$,

$P<.001$, 1-year follow-up). Individuals with predominantly simple-partial seizures, including those with mostly auras, achieved the greatest clinical benefit (see **Fig. 3**). Overall, these patients were significantly more likely to become responders by 1 year than those with other seizure types (OR, 1.37; 95% CI, 1.04–1.81, $P = .025$). In contrast, the lowest rates of clinical response were seen among patients with either primary generalized or secondarily generalized tonic-clonic seizures (see **Fig. 3**). Together, generalized tonic-clonic seizures were negatively predictive of clinical response to VNS at 1 year with an OR of 0.77 (95% CI, 0.63–0.93; $P = .008$). Patients with other generalized seizure types, including atonic drop attacks, responded to therapy in more than 57% of cases by 1 year (see **Fig. 3**). These results suggest that patients with predominantly

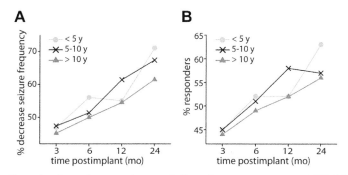

Fig. 2. A longer duration of epilepsy is somewhat predictive of poorer response to VNS. (*A*) Median percentage decrease in seizure frequency at 3, 6, 12, and 24 months after VNS implantation compared with preoperative baseline, stratified by duration of epilepsy. (*B*) Percentage of patients who clinically responded to VNS, achieving a decrease of 50% or more in seizure frequency after VNS compared with baseline. Patients with more than 10 years of seizures responded to VNS less frequently than those with less than 10 years of epilepsy, although this trend did not reach statistical significance ($P = .053$ at 12 months). N at 3, 6, 12, and 24 months are 469, 298, 251, and 79 for duration of less than 5 years; 871, 589, 500, and 192 for duration of 5 to 10 years; and 2789, 1913, 1732, and 759 for duration of more than 10 years.

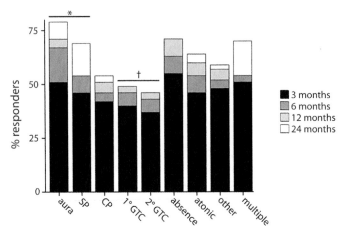

Fig. 3. Response to VNS therapy varies by predominant seizure type. Data shown are percentage of patients who clinically responded to VNS at 3, 6, 12, and 24 months after surgery, with results stratified by predominant preoperative seizure type. Individuals with multiple seizure types did not display a single predominant seizure semiology. Responders achieved a decrease of 50% or more in seizure frequency after VNS compared with preoperative baseline. Significantly higher (*asterisk*) or significantly lower (*dagger*) responder rates compared with individuals with all other seizure types are indicated ($P<.05$). N at 3, 6, 12, and 24 months are 76, 55, 49, and 19 for aura-only; 300, 212, 182, and 86 for SP; 2020, 1376, 1241, and 531 for CP; 484, 316, 275, and 124 for 1° GTC; 325, 238, 214, and 97 for 2° GTC; 284, 196, 158, and 59 for absence, 225, 139, 142, and 45 for atonic; 399, 269, 229, and 73 for other; and 370, 239, 208, and 70 for multiple seizure types. CP, complex partial; 1° GTC, primary generalized tonic clonic; 2° GTC, secondarily generalized tonic clonic; SP, simple partial.

partial seizures, particularly simple-partial seizures and auras, respond most favorably to VNS, whereas those with generalized tonic-clonic seizures respond least favorably. Nevertheless, 46% to 49% of patients with predominantly generalized tonic-clonic seizures still achieve a decrease of 50% or more in seizures after 1 year of VNS.

We also analyzed whether or not patients with Lennox-Gastaut syndrome and other epileptic encephalopathies, disorders accounting for some of the most debilitating cases of epilepsy, responded to VNS differently compared with other individuals. At 1 year of therapy, 314 individuals with epileptic encephalopathy achieved a median decrease of 66% in seizure frequency and a response rate of 61% compared with a seizure decrease of only 55% and a response rate of 52% in 2384 patients without this diagnosis ($\chi^2 = 7.9$, $P = .006$, comparing response rates). The diagnosis of epileptic encephalopathy was significantly predictive of a favorable response (OR, 1.41; 95% CI, 1.11–1.79; $P = .005$), suggesting better efficacy of VNS in this patient population.

DISCUSSION

Approximately 30% of patients with epilepsy are refractory to medical therapy, and many of these individuals are poor candidates for surgical resection because of multifocal seizure origin or eloquence near epileptic foci.[1,2] VNS was approved

by the US FDA as an adjunctive treatment of intractable epilepsy in 1997, but its approval was limited to individuals aged 12 years and more with partial epilepsy.[3–5] Disagreement persists regarding the efficacy of VNS for epilepsy and about which patient populations respond best to therapy. In this article, we report the largest, to our knowledge, retrospective analysis of VNS efficacy in patients with epilepsy. We stratified seizure outcomes from a large patient registry by various potential predictors of response. Across all patients, we observed a progressive clinical response to VNS during the first 24 months of treatment. After 3 months of treatment, 44% of individuals experienced 50% or more fewer seizures compared with preoperative baseline, with a median decrease in seizure frequency of 46%. However, at 2-year follow-up, these outcomes improved to a patient response rate of 54% and a reduction in seizure frequency of 62%. We also found that patients aged 18 years or less, including children younger than 6 years, achieved a higher rate of clinical response to VNS therapy than adults at 1 year and that individuals with shorter duration of epilepsy responded more favorably than those with a seizure history of more than 10 years. Both these findings suggest that earlier intervention with VNS may lead to improved efficacy and should thus be considered in the appropriate patient. Furthermore, these data suggest that despite its initial approval for adults and adolescents, VNS likely provides similar or superior seizure reduction in children and should be considered in pediatric patients.

We also examined various seizure types as potential predictors of response to VNS. Patients with predominantly focal seizures, particularly simple-partial seizures and auras, achieved the highest rates of clinical response (54%–71% at 1 year, 69%–79% at 2 years). However, only 46% to 49% of patients with generalized tonic-clonic seizures had responded favorably at 1- and 2-year follow-up evaluations. This disparity is perhaps not surprising given the original indication of VNS for partial epilepsy syndromes only. However, considering the significant morbidity associated with generalized tonic-clonic seizures, a likelihood of more than 45% of reducing seizures by 50% or more may make VNS a desirable option for some patients with these seizure types as well. Furthermore, patients with generalized seizure types other than tonic-clonic seizures responded more favorably to therapy ($\geq$57% response rate) by 1 year. We found that patients with other epileptic encephalopathies such as Lennox-Gastaut syndrome responded particularly well to VNS therapy. These are particularly debilitating epileptic syndromes in which VNS can be considered to reduce the burden of recurrent, generalized, and multifocal seizures.[12,13]

Although adverse effects related to VNS therapy were not studied, they represent important considerations in making treatment decisions. In 3 large prospective studies, hoarseness or change in voice was the most common adverse effect, reported by 37% to 55% of patients.[9,10,14] Cough, paresthesia, pain, dyspnea, and headache are also sometimes reported. Infection has been reported by investigators in 4% to 6% of implants, often necessitating device explantation,[10,14] with an infection rate of 1.7% over the past 3 years recorded by the manufacturer (data provided by Cyberonics, Inc). Asystole was described in 5 early cases of VNS,[3] and the device manufacturer has recorded 59 reports of intraoperative asystole (0.76 events per 1000 implants) and 21 cases of postoperative asystole (0.06 events per 1000 patient-years) from July 1997 to March 2011 (data provided by Cyberonics, Inc), although it remains unclear if stimulation directly caused these serious occurrences.

It is also necessary to recognize the limitations of VNS therapy in epilepsy to guide treatment discussions and manage expectations of both patients and physicians. Patients may be counseled that although overall VNS has been shown to reduce seizure frequency by 50% or more in more than half of the treated patients, complete seizure freedom is rare, and some patients experience no improvement in symptoms. Varied response rates among individuals of different ages, epilepsy duration, and seizures types, as examined in this study, should also be considered. Furthermore, an appreciation of the delayed clinical benefit often associated with VNS is important during the first few months of treatment. Nevertheless, given the debilitating effects of recurrent seizures on a patient's neuropsychological profile and quality of life, VNS should be considered in those who have failed medical therapy and are not candidates for potential cure by resective surgery.

It is important to recognize the limitations of the present study. Given the nature of a retrospective patient registry analysis, we cannot independently ascertain the validity of clinical data submitted by individual physicians. The possibility of selection bias in reporting also cannot be excluded. This uncertainty would be best addressed in a single large prospective series. Nevertheless, the strength of this evaluation lies in the ability to pool an exceptionally large number of cases that would be difficult to achieve even in a multi-institutional trial. The long-term clinical outcomes of VNS are not fully known and must be scrutinized going forward, particularly given the progressive increase in efficacy observed with VNS during the first 2 years of therapy.

SUMMARY

Through a retrospective review of a patient registry, we examined the largest population of patients with epilepsy treated with VNS therapy in the published literature, to our knowledge. Across all patients, seizure frequency decreased progressively from 46% fewer seizures at 3 months to a reduction of 62% at 2 years of treatment. More than half of the patients responded well at 1-year follow-up, achieving a decrease of 50% or more in seizure frequency. Age of 18 years or more, epilepsy duration of 10 or more years, and a predominance of partial seizures predicted a more favorable clinical response, and patients with epileptic encephalopathies such as Lennox-Gastaut syndrome received increased benefit compared with other individuals. Given the debilitating effects of epilepsy on patient quality of life, VNS should be considered in those who have failed medical therapy and are not candidates for resective surgery.

REFERENCES

1. Mohanraj R, Brodie MJ. Diagnosing refractory epilepsy: response to sequential treatment schedules. Eur J Neurol 2006;13:277–82.

2. Jehi LE, Silveira DC, Bingaman W, et al. Temporal lobe epilepsy surgery failures: predictors of seizure recurrence, yield of reevaluation, and outcome following reoperation. J Neurosurg 2010;113: 1186–94.

3. Ben-Menachem E. Vagus-nerve stimulation for the treatment of epilepsy. Lancet Neurol 2002;1: 477–82.

4. Chang EF, Barbaro NM. Nonresective epilepsy surgery. Epilepsia 2010;51(Suppl 1):87–9.

5. Schachter SC, Saper CB. Vagus nerve stimulation. Epilepsia 1998;39:677–86.

6. Chase MH, Nakamura Y, Clemente CD, et al. Afferent vagal stimulation: neurographic correlates of induced EEG synchronization and desynchronization. Brain Res 1967;5:236–49.

7. Henry TR. Therapeutic mechanisms of vagus nerve stimulation. Neurology 2002;59:S3–14.

8. Koo B. EEG changes with vagus nerve stimulation. J Clin Neurophysiol 2001;18:434–41.

9. Ben-Menachem E, Manon-Espaillat R, Ristanovic R, et al. Vagus nerve stimulation for treatment of partial seizures: 1. A controlled study of effect on seizures. First International Vagus Nerve Stimulation Study Group. Epilepsia 1994;35:616–26.

10. Handforth A, DeGiorgio CM, Schachter SC, et al. Vagus nerve stimulation therapy for partial-onset seizures: a randomized active-control trial. Neurology 1998;51:48–55.

11. Amar AP, Apuzzo ML, Liu CY. Vagus nerve stimulation therapy after failed cranial surgery for intractable epilepsy: results from the vagus nerve stimulation therapy patient outcome registry. Neurosurgery 2004;55:1086–93.

12. Arzimanoglou A, French J, Blume WT, et al. Lennox-Gastaut syndrome: a consensus approach on diagnosis, assessment, management, and trial methodology. Lancet Neurol 2009;8:82–93.

13. Cersosimo RO, Bartuluchi M, De Los Santos C, et al. Vagus nerve stimulation: effectiveness and tolerability in patients with epileptic encephalopathies. Childs Nerv Syst 2011;27:787–92.

14. DeGiorgio CM, Schachter SC, Handforth A, et al. Prospective long-term study of vagus nerve stimulation for the treatment of refractory seizures. Epilepsia 2000;41:1195–200.

Trigeminal Nerve Stimulation: Seminal Animal and Human Studies for Epilepsy and Depression

Christopher M. DeGiorgio, MD[a],*, Erika E. Fanselow, PhD[b],
Lara M. Schrader, MD[a], Ian A. Cook, MD[c]

KEYWORDS

- Trigeminal nerve stimulation • Epilepsy • Depression
- Drug resistant epilepsy

Epilepsy affects 3 million Americans, of whom 1 million (30%) have drug-resistant epilepsy.[1,2,3,4] Drug-resistant epilepsy frequently leads to unemployment, injuries, and sudden death.[1,2,3,4] Likewise, major depression is a significant public health problem, affecting more than 17 million American adults, a significant number of whom are persistently ill despite multiple trials of antidepressant medications.[5,6,7] Given the side effects of drug therapy for both conditions (eg, sedation, cognitive impairment, behavioral side effects, weight gain and metabolic syndrome, risk for allergies, and suicide), there is a need for alternative nondrug therapies for both epilepsy and depression.

There is growing interest in neuromodulation for depression and epilepsy, including vagus nerve stimulation (VNS), repetitive transcranial magnetic stimulation (rTMS), and deep brain stimulation (DBS) as alternatives to failed drug therapy.[8,9,10,11,12,13,14] These approaches are expensive, have modest efficacy, and can be surgically invasive. Trigeminal nerve stimulation (TNS) is an emerging neuromodulation therapy with unique advantages: it can be delivered externally, bilaterally, and at low cost.[15,16] Response during a trial of external TNS can be used to evaluate potential surgical candidates before an implantable stimulation device is inserted.[15,16] This article evaluates the anatomy of the trigeminal nerve, presents animal data, and summarizes recent developments in the application of TNS in drug-resistant epilepsy and major depressive disorder.[15,16,17]

ANATOMY OF THE TRIGEMINAL NERVE

The trigeminal nerve is the largest cranial nerve (fifth or CN V), and has extensive connections with brainstem and other brain structures.[18,19,20,21] The trigeminal nerve has 3 major sensory branches over the face, all of which are bilateral (**Fig. 1**).[18] These branches pass through 3 foramens in the skull, just lateral to the midline.[22] The nerves within these foramens also supply sensation over the facial structures, and project to the main trigeminal ganglion at the base of the skull.[18] The ophthalmic branch (V1) is ideally placed to allow bilateral stimulation using a single paired electrode placed over the forehead. **Fig. 2** details the anatomy of the ophthalmic division of the trigeminal nerve.

Disclosure: See last page of article.
[a] Department of Neurology, David Geffen School of Medicine at UCLA, 710 Westwood Plaza, Los Angeles, CA 90095, USA
[b] Department of Neurobiology, University of Pittsburgh School of Medicine, Pittsburgh, PA, USA
[c] Depression Research and Clinic Program, Semel Institute for Neuroscience and Human Behavior at UCLA, 760 Westwood Plaza, Los Angeles, CA 90095, USA
* Corresponding author.
E-mail address: cmd@mednet.ucla.edu

Neurosurg Clin N Am 22 (2011) 449–456
doi:10.1016/j.nec.2011.07.001
1042-3680/11/$ – see front matter © 2011 Elsevier Inc. All rights reserved.

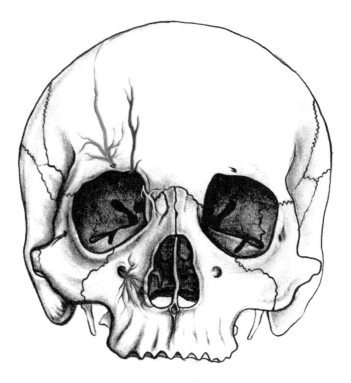

Fig. 1. Anatomy of the cutaneous branches of the trigeminal nerve: V1 and V2 are shown. (*Courtesy o* Emerson.)

The trigeminal ganglion, located in the Meckel cave (cavum trigeminale), projects to the trigeminal nucleus, which has reciprocal projections to the nucleus tractus solitarius (NTS), locus coeruleus, and the reticular formation, structures that play an important role in inhibition of seizures.[18,19,20,21] Evidence from animals indicates that stimulation of the trigeminal nerve and its related structures inhibit seizures.[17,23,24,25,26] NTS stimulation was investigated in a cat model of epilepsy.[23] NTS stimulation delayed the onset of overt seizures induced by chronic amygdala stimulation (an animal model commonly used to produce chronic epilepsy).[23] The latency to the development of seizures was significantly delayed, and many animals never developed the expected seizures.[23] Overall, intermittent NTS stimulation prolonged or inhibited the onset of kindled seizures.[23] The trigeminal nucleus also has extensive projections to locus coeruleus and midbrain periaqueductal gray, structures involved in the production of the catecholamine neurotransmitters epinephrine and norepinephrine.[25,26] Stimulation of the locus coeruleus suppresses epileptic discharges induced by cobalt and penicillin, agents used to provoke seizures in animals.[27] The locus coeruleus plays a central role in the anticonvulsant effect of VNS and, given the projections of the trigeminal nerve to the vagus

nerve via the reticular formation, the locus c leus may share a common role in the effica both VNS and TNS.[28]

Based on animal data linking stimulati central trigeminal pathways to an antiep effect, Fanselow and colleagues[17] initiated s of TNS using a rat model of epilepsy, and DeG and colleagues[8,15,16] initiated phase I c studies of infraorbital and supraorbital TN intractable seizures in humans. In this reviev results of these seminal studies will be prese

ANIMAL STUDIES

Cranial nerve stimulation has been used for than a decade to reduce seizure activity in pa with epilepsy. Specifically, the technique o received US Food and Drug Administ approval in 1997 and has been implemen tens of thousands of patients.[8,9,29] Howeve mechanisms by which VNS alleviates seizu responsive patients are not well understooc not all patients are candidates for, or respc to, this therapy.[30] Further, it was not prev clear whether the seizure-reduction effect c was specific to the vagus nerve, or wheth effect could be generalized to other cranial n

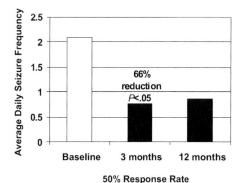

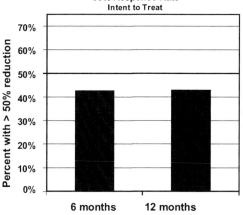

Fig. 2. Pilot feasibility trial of TNS for epilepsy. Change in average daily seizure frequency (*left*). Note that, at 3 months, the reduction in seizures was 66% of the initial therapeutic threshold (Intent to treat), *P*<.05.

Therefore, in the laboratory of Dr M.A.L. Nicolelis in the Department of Neurobiology at Duke University, Fanselow and colleagues[17] tested whether stimulation of another cranial nerve, the trigeminal nerve, could exert anticonvulsant effects in awake rats.

METHODS FOR STIMULATING THE TRIGEMINAL NERVE IN RATS

Initial animal studies of TNS were performed in awake, adult rats using the pentylenetetrazole-induced seizure model.[17] Rats were surgically implanted with arrays of chronic, indwelling electrodes in layer V of the somatosensory cortex and in the somatosensory thalamus.[17] These electrodes allowed for local field potential (LFP) recordings at 16 sites within each recording target. Seizures were initiated using intraperitoneal injection of pentylenetetrazole (40 mg/kg).[17] Injection of this agent induced generalized tonic-clonic seizures with a duration of about 4 seconds and a frequency of 4 per minute for approximately 2 hours.[17]

To reliably activate the trigeminal nerve in awake animals, a nerve cuff electrode, constructed in-house, was implanted around the infraorbital branch of the trigeminal nerve.[17] The nerve cuff electrode contained 2 platinum bands between which current was passed to activate fibers in the infraorbital nerve.[17] This branch of the trigeminal nerve carries somatosensory input from the whiskers on the face of the rat to the trigeminal ganglion, which subsequently projects to the trigeminal brainstem nuclei.[17] These nuclei project to the ventroposterior medial nucleus of the thalamus, which sends afferents to the primary somatosensory cortex.[18]

In these studies, trains of trigeminal stimuli were presented at varying frequencies and amplitudes.[17] Stimulus trains were presented using a continuous duty cycle of 1 minute on to 1 minute off. Seizures observed in the LFP recordings were quantified in 3 ways: (1) number of seizures, (2) seizure duration, and (3) integrated seizure activity, a measure of overall seizure activity calculated by integrating the absolute value of the LFP signals.[17]

REDUCTION OF SEIZURES IN ANIMALS DURING TNS

When TNS was applied during pentylenetetrazole administration, seizure activity was reduced in the thalamus and neocortex according to all 3 measures of seizure prevalence.[17] At a stimulus frequency of greater than 100 Hz and a stimulus intensity of 11 mA, a seizure reduction of 78% was observed across all animals.[17] In addition to a reduction in electrographic measures of seizures, as measured in the cortical and thalamic LFPs, the behavioral characteristics of the pentylenetetrazole-induced seizures (clonic jerking of the body and forelimbs) were concomitantly reduced.[17] Thus, the seizure-reduction effect was not specific solely to the somatosensory regions of the thalamus and neocortex.[17]

The seizure-reduction effect was dependent on both stimulus frequency and stimulus intensity.[17] It was necessary to stimulate at greater than 50 Hz to observe a reduction in seizure activity.[17] Increasing stimulus frequency to more than 100 Hz showed no improvement in seizure reduction and, with frequencies less than 50 Hz, there was a trend toward increased seizure duration, peaking at a stimulus frequency of 10 Hz.[17] Seizure reduction increased with increasing current levels, presumably because higher current levels activated more fibers in the stimulated infraorbital branch of the trigeminal nerve.[17] TNS had no discernable effect on heart rate, and animals did not show distress at the levels of stimulation used in these studies.[17]

These initial experiments showed that TNS was effective at reducing pentylenetetrazole-induced seizures in awake animals. We were also interested in 2 other aspects of TNS efficacy against seizures. The first of these was the use of bilateral TNS, and the second was seizure-triggered stimulation.

Efficacy of Bilateral TNS

Unlike VNS, in which typically only the left vagus nerve is stimulated to avoid cardiac side effects, TNS can readily be applied to both trigeminal nerves simultaneously.[8,9,15,16] However, it was not known whether this would improve the efficacy of TNS or whether unilateral stimulation of the trigeminal nerve was sufficient to elicit the full seizure-reduction effect of TNS. Therefore, nerve cuff electrodes were implanted bilaterally on each of the infraorbital nerves along with indwelling electrodes in each of the primary somatosensory cortices.[17] Each infraorbital nerve was stimulated individually and then both nerves were stimulated simultaneously.[17] When both infraorbital nerves were stimulated simultaneously, there was a decrease in the current required to achieve maximal seizure reduction.[17] That is, with unilateral TNS, a stimulus intensity of 11 mA was required to achieve 75% seizure reduction, whereas with bilateral stimulation the same degree of seizure reduction was accomplished with 7 mA of current presented to each nerve simultaneously.[17] This result suggests that the effects of TNS increase with multiple nerve stimulation sites, which has implications for the optimization of TNS application in patient populations.[17] The electrographic (and behavioral) seizure-reduction effects were identical for each side stimulated (ie, either contralateral or ipsilateral to the neocortical recording site).[17] This is further evidence that the effects of TNS involve more than just the brain regions directly targeted by the trigeminal nerve.[17]

Closed-loop Seizure-triggered TNS

An open question about cranial nerve stimulation was whether it was better to provide stimulation on a continuous on-off duty cycle or to apply responsive stimulation only when a seizure was detected. Such a closed-loop paradigm required the development of a seizure-detection algorithm capable of detecting a seizure and promptly triggering TNS. In conjunction with Ashlan P. Reid in the Department of Biomedical Engineering at Duke University, a seizure detector was developed that triggered TNS when the LFP signal increased

to more than a manually set voltage threshold.[17] When such activity was detected in the LFP, 500 millisecond trains of 500-microsecond pulses were delivered until the aberrant LFP activity was no longer detected.[17] When unilateral TNS was provided in this seizure-triggered manner, it successfully stopped seizure activity, in an average of 529 milliseconds after seizure onset.[17] This seizure-reduction effect was not observed when TNS was initiated manually after a seizure had been underway for more than 10 seconds (Fanselow, Reid, and Nicolelis, unpublished observations, 2010), so it therefore seemed to be critical to provide the stimulation early in a seizure episode. These results showed that TNS could successfully be applied in a closed-loop, seizure-triggered manner. This finding has implications for the mechanism(s) by which TNS reduces seizure activity. It is likely that, in humans, a more sophisticated seizure-detection algorithm would be required for implementation of a closed-loop stimulation paradigm, but these results serve as a proof of principle for seizure-triggered TNS.

Potential Mechanisms of TNS Seizure-reduction Effects

The mechanisms by which any type of cranial nerve stimulation reduces seizure activity are poorly understood. Multiple studies have suggested that a component of the effect of VNS on seizures is caused by involvement of the neuromodulators released from brainstem nuclei or their downstream targets. For example, Krahl and colleagues[28] showed that lesions of the locus coeruleus, the noradrenergic nucleus of the brainstem, blocked the seizure-suppression effects of VNS. Recent evidence for the involvement of norepinephrine was obtained by Raedt and colleagues[31] who showed that norepinephrine levels in the hippocampus increased during VNS. Whether noradrenergic effects are also present during TNS is not yet known. In addition, the reticular activating system, including the reticular formation of the brainstem, has been implicated in reducing seizure activity, primarily because stimulation of this region is known to desynchronize firing in the neocortex.[32]

It is likely that there are multiple mechanisms by which cranial nerve stimulation, including TNS, exerts its effects on the brain. Evidence for this comes from the different time scales on which cranial nerve stimulation can be effective. First, as discussed earlier, seizure-triggered TNS was able to abort seizures on a rapid time scale, suggesting that TNS can have immediate effects on seizure activity.[17] In support of this, there is evidence that neuronal firing is suppressed during TNS in rats as soon as the nerve stimulation begins.[33] Second, in humans, VNS and TNS are typically provided on a continuous fixed-duty cycle, and, in animal studies, it has been shown that there is a period of increased seizure threshold after termination of each On cycle.[17,34] Therefore, there may also be effects of cranial nerve stimulation that last from tens of seconds to minutes and outlast the period of nerve stimulation. In addition, there seem to be long-term effects of cranial nerve stimulation, in which seizure frequency and severity are observed to decrease in the course of months to years.[8,35,36,37] This finding suggests that TNS could potentially cause long-term alterations in the brain that could depend on genetically mediated changes in brain function, as has been shown for VNS.[8,35,36] None of these seizure-reduction mechanisms are mutually exclusive, and they could operate concurrently to reduce seizure activity.

CONCLUSIONS FROM ANIMAL STUDIES OF TNS, AND FUTURE DIRECTIONS

Animal studies showed that TNS was effective for reducing seizure activity, that bilateral trigeminal stimulation was more effective than unilateral stimulation, and that TNS was effective when delivered in a closed-loop, seizure-triggered paradigm. These studies prepared the way for subsequent studies of TNS in human subjects, as discussed later. Future animal studies will investigate the cellular-level/circuit-level mechanisms by which TNS exerts its effects, and, based on this information, explore ways to optimize stimulus parameters to maximize the seizure-reduction capabilities of TNS in patients with epilepsy.

Pilot Feasibility Trials in Humans with Epilepsy and Depression

Epilepsy

Beginning in 2001, subjects with severe epilepsy with a minimum of 3 seizures per month were enrolled in an open-label pilot feasibility study of external infraorbital and supraorbital TNS in Los Angeles (CA). Thirteen subjects entered a 1-month pretreatment baseline and, after 1 month, were treated with TNS with a duty cycle of up to 30 seconds on to 30 seconds off.[15,16]

Subjects were initiated with infraorbital TNS, but external infraorbital TNS proved awkward. Subjects were then converted to receiving TNS delivered via supraorbital electrodes, which allowed for bilateral stimulation using a sustainable and well-tolerated platform. Initial studies focused safety and feasibility issues, such as on the effect

of TNS on pain, stimulation intensity studies, and the effects of TNS on heart rate and blood pressure. TNS was well tolerated. Side effects were infrequent and mild, but included skin irritation, which improved by reducing stimulation to 12 to 16 hours/d, or through application of 1% hydrocortisone cream.[15,16] Tingling, forehead pressure, and headache were reported, but improved with reduction of current.[15,16] Extensive monitoring of pulse and blood pressure were performed acutely after initial exposure to TNS, and chronically for at least 1 year.[16] No effect was identified on electrocardiograph, heart rate, or systolic or diastolic blood pressure.[16] With regard to therapeutic effects, at 3 months, the mean seizure frequency was reduced by 66%, from a pretreatment baseline of 2.1, to 0.71 seizures/d ($P<.05$).[16] At 12 months, the mean seizure frequency was 0.86 seizures/d (59% reduction, $P = .058$).[16] Five subjects experienced greater than 50% reduction at 6 and 12 months, and 1 subject had greater than 90% reduction.[16] Replacing the electrodes daily, TNS can be used for years, and some patients have used the device for up to 5 years[16] **Figs. 1** and **2** shows the acute and long-term efficacy at 3 and 12 months, as well as responder rates at 6 and 12 months of long-term follow-up. In this pilot trial, responder rates using intent-to-treat analysis (which does not inflate response rates caused by dropouts) showed efficacy that favorably compares with responder rates of VNS, DBS, and renal nerve stimulation. This finding requires confirmation in future controlled clinical trials.[8,9,10] In light of the positive results from the pilot feasibility study, and the absence of any adverse effect of TNS on heart rate and blood pressure, a randomized, phase II, controlled clinical trial of high versus low TNS was begun at 2 sites in Los Angeles (CA) to evaluate TNS in double-blind controlled conditions. Fifty subjects were enrolled. Initial results are promising, and the study results should be available by early 2012, and will inform a larger pivotal trial of TNS.

Major Depression

Given the anatomy of the trigeminal nerve, and its projection to structures associated with mood regulation, Drs Lara Schrader and Ian Cook initiated an exploratory study of TNS in major depression. Five adults ages 31 to 59 years with nonpsychotic unipolar major depressive disorder were studied in an 8-week open-label outpatient trial at University of California, Los Angeles.[38] Entry criteria included duration of illness of at least 4 months, persistent depressive symptoms despite at least 1 antidepressant at acceptable doses during the current episode, pharmacotherapy

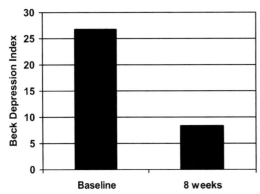

Fig. 3. TNS in major depression. Results from the First Pilot Feasibility Trial. The change in Beck Depression Index was significant: 2-tailed *t*-test, *P* = .0004. (*Data from* Cook IA, DeGiorgio CM, Miller PM, et al. Noninvasive neuromodulation with trigeminal nerve stimulation: a novel treatment for major depressive disorder. Poster presented at the NCDEU Annual Meeting. Boca Raton (FL), June 14–17, 2010.)

with at least 1 antidepressant in at least 6 weeks during the current episode, and concomitant use of at least 1 antidepressant at study entry.[38] All had prominent depressive symptoms, with a mean entry score on the 17-item Hamilton Depression Rating Scale (HDRS-17) of 16.2 (standard deviation [SD]3.3).[38] Subjects placed stimulating electrodes over the supraorbital branches of the trigeminal nerve for at least 8 hours per day (primarily while asleep), with current adjusted to maximal comfortable levels.[38]

Overall, TNS for major depression was well tolerated. No serious side effects occurred in the 8-week treatment period, and no adverse effect on blood pressure or heart rate was detected. Responses on the Beck Depression Inventory (BDI) declined significantly, from a baseline mean BDI of 26.8 (SD 8.1) to 8.4 (4.9) at 8 weeks (2-tail *t*-test, *P* = .0004). **Fig. 3**[38] summarizes the acute response in the 8-week acute treatment period. Depressive symptoms improved whether assessed with a self-rated (BDI) or clinician-rated (HDRS-17) instrument.[38] Overall, the preliminary data indicate an early and robust response of TNS for major depression.[38] These findings are now being confirmed in a larger cohort, and a randomized, phase II, double-blind trial is underway to evaluate the efficacy of TNS using a double-blind controlled design.

SUMMARY

TNS is a new method to treat both epilepsy and major depression. The unique ability to stimulate bilaterally, extracranially, and noninvasively

represents a significant advantage to existing neuromodulation therapies. In humans thus far the technique has been applied noninvasively, termed external TNS. If external TNS is effective, it could lead to the development of a more convenient implantable device for patients who are responders to external TNS. The potential to predict responders to an implantable TNS devise using noninvasive means would be a significant benefit compared with other currently available implantable neuromodulatory devices.

We are completing O^{15} positron emission tomography studies, which will shed light on which structures are being activated or inhibited by TNS. This work will advance the understanding of mechanisms of action for this novel neuromodulation therapy. In addition, phase II randomized clinical trials are near completion for both epilepsy and depression, and larger phase III trials are in the planning stages. TNS represents an exciting addition to existing invasive neuromodulation therapies for epilepsy and depression.

DISCLOSURES

This work is supported by generous donations to the UCLA Department of Neurology by James and Beverly Peters, Robert and Linda Brill, Mark and Terry Jacoby, the Salter, Lester, Lagermeir families, Mrs Elsie Johnson, and through the generosity of an anonymous donor, and Mr and Mrs Dietel Hopps. Additional support was provided by the Joanne and George Miller and Family Endowment in Depression Research at the UCLA Brain Research Institute. Drs DeGiorgio, Cook, and Schrader are among the inventors of patents assigned to the Regents of the University of California and exclusively licensed to NeuroSigma, Inc. In addition, Dr DeGiorgio discloses grant support from the Epilepsy Therapy Project, Epilepsy Foundation of America, Milken Family Foundation, Boston Scientific/Advanced Bionics, and the NIH. Dr Cook discloses that, in the past 5 years, he has served as an advisor or consultant to Ascend Media, Bristol-Myers Squibb, Cyberonics, Neuronetics, NeuroSigma, Scale Venture Partners, US Department of Defense, and US Department of Justice; has received grant/research support from Aspect Medical Systems/Covidien, Cyberonics, Lilly, Neuronetics, NIH, Novartis, Pfizer, Seaside Therapeutics, Sepracor; and has been compensated to speak on behalf of Bristol-Myers Squibb, Medical Education Speakers Network, Neuronetics, NeuroSigma, and Wyeth. He has accepted stock options in NeuroSigma. Dr Schrader and Dr Fanselow have no additional disclosures.

REFERENCES

1. Begley CE, Famulari M, Annegers J, et al. The cost of epilepsy in the United States: an estimate from population-based clinical and survey data. Epilepsia 2000;41:342.
2. Weibe S, Blume WT, Girvin JP, et al. A randomized, controlled trial of surgery for temporal lobe epilepsy. N Engl J Med 2001;345:311–8.
3. Sperling MR, Feldman H, Kinman J, et al. Seizure control and mortality in epilepsy. Ann Neurol 1999; 46:45–50.
4. Cockerell OC, Johnson AL, Sander JW. Mortality from epilepsy: results from a prospective population-based study. Lancet 1994;344:918–21.
5. Kessler RC, Berglund P, Demler O, et al. The epidemiology of major depressive disorder: results from the National Comorbidity Survey Replication (NCS-R). JAMA 2003;289:3095–105.
6. Rush AJ, Trivedi MH, Wisniewski SR, et al. Acute and longer-term outcomes in depressed outpatients requiring one or several treatment steps: A STAR*D report. Am J Psychiatry 2006;163:1905–17.
7. Gaynes BN, Warden D, Trivedi MH, et al. What did STAR*D teach us? Results from a large-scale, practical, clinical trial for patients with depression. Psychiatr Serv 2009;60:1439–45.
8. DeGiorgio CM, Schachter SC, Handforth A, et al. Prospective long-term study of vagus nerve stimulation for the treatment of refractory seizures. Epilepsia 2000;41:1195–2000.
9. Handforth A, DeGiorgio C, Schachter S. Vagus nerve stimulation therapy for partial-onset seizures: a randomized active-control trial. Neurology 1998; 51:48–55.
10. Fisher R, Salanova V, Witt T, et al. Electrical stimulation of the anterior nucleus of thalamus for treatment of refractory epilepsy. Epilepsia 2010;51:899–908.
11. Skarpass TL, Morrell M. Intracranial stimulation therapy for epilepsy. Neurotherapeutics 2009;6: 238–43.
12. Marangell LB, Martinez M, Jurdi RA, et al. Neurostimulation therapies in depression: a review of new modalities. Acta Pscyhiatr Scan 2007;116:174–81.
13. George MS, Wassermann EM, Post RM. Transcranial magnetic stimulation: a neuropsychiatric tool for the 21st century. J Neuropsychiatry Clin Neurosci 1996; 8:373–82.
14. Mayberg HS, Lozano AM, Voon V, et al. Deep brain stimulation for treatment-resistant depression. Neuron 2005;45:651–60.
15. DeGiorgio CM, Shewmon DA, Whitehurst T. Pilot feasibility study of trigeminal nerve stimulation for epilepsy. A proof of concept trial. Epilepsia 2006; 47:1213–5.
16. DeGiorgio C, Murray D, Markovic D Whitehurst T. Trigeminal nerve stimulation for epilepsy: long-term feasibility and efficacy. Neurology 2009;72:936–8, 19273830.
17. Fanselow EE, Reid A, Nicolelis AL. Reduction of pentylenetetrazole induced seizure activity in awake rats by seizure-triggered trigeminal nerve stimulation. J Neurosci 2000;20:8160–8.
18. Anatomy: A Regional Atlas of the Human Body, 5th edition, 2006. Lippincott, Williams and Wilkins; 1997.
19. Caous CA, de Sousa Buck H, Lindsey CJ. Neuronal connections of the paratrigeminal nucleus. Auton Neurosci 2001;94:14–24.
20. Grzanna R, Chee WK, Akeyson EW. Noradrenergic projections to brainstem nuclei: evidence for differential projections from noradrenergic subgroups. J Comp Neurol 1987;263:76–91.
21. Krout KE, Belzer RE, Loewy AD. Brainstem projections to midline and intra-laminar thalamic nuclei of the rat. J Comp Neurol 2002;448:53–101.
22. Cutright B, Quillopa N, Schubert W. An anthropometric analysis of the key foramina for maxillofacial surgery. J Oral Maxillofac Surg 2010;61:354–7.
23. Magdaleno-Madrigal VM, Valdes Cruz A, Martinez Vargas D, et al. Effect of electrical stimulation of the nucleus of the solitary tract on the development of electrical amygdaloid kindling in the cat. Epilepsia 2002;43:964.
24. Walker BR, Easton A, Gale K. Regulation of limbic motor seizures by GABA and glutamate transmission in nucleus tractus solitarius. Epilepsia 1999; 40:1051–7.
25. Sasa M, Ohno Y, Nabatame H, et al. Effects of L-threo-dops, an L-noradrenaline precursor, on locus coeruleus originating neurons in spinal trigeminal nucleus. Brain Res 1987;420:157–61.
26. Hoskin KL, Bulmer DC, Lasalandra M. Fos expression in the midbrain peri-aqueductal grey after trigeminal-vascular stimulation. J Anat 2001;198:29–35.
27. Weiss GK, Lewis J, Jimenez-Rivera C, et al. Antikindling effects of locus coeruleus stimulation: mediation by ascending noradrenergic projections. Exp Neurol 1990;108:136–40.
28. Krahl SE, Clark K, Smith D, et al. Locus coeruleus lesions suppress the seizure-attenuating effects of vagus nerve stimulation. Epilepsia 1998;39:709–14.
29. Lulic D, Ahmadian A, Baaj AA, et al. Vagus nerve stimulation. Neurosurg Focus 2009;27:E5.
30. Ghaemi K, Elsharkawy AE, Schulz R, et al. Vagus nerve stimulation: outcome and predictors of seizure freedom in long-term follow-up. Seizure 2010;19: 264–8.
31. Raedt R, Clinckers R, Mollet L, et al. Increased hippocampal noradrenaline is a biomarker for efficacy of vagus nerve stimulation in a limbic seizure model. J Neurochem 2011;117:461–9.
32. Moruzzi G, Magoun HW. Brain stem reticular formation and activation of the EEG. Electroencephalogr Clin Neurophysiol 1949;1:455–73.

33. Fanselow E, Noel D. Reduction of neocortical neuronal firing by therapeutic trigeminal nerve stimulation. Presented at the American Epilepsy Society Annual Meeting. San Antonio (TX), December 4, 2010.

34. Takaya M, Terry WJ, Naritoku DK. Vagus nerve stimulation induces a sustained anticonvulsant effect. Epilepsia 1996;37:1111–6.

35. Morris GL 3rd, Mueller WM. Long-term treatment with vagus nerve stimulation in patients with refractory epilepsy. The Vagus Nerve Stimulation Study Group E01-E05. Neurology 1999;53:1731–5.

36. Uthman BM, Reichl AM, Dean JC, et al. Effectiveness of vagus nerve stimulation in epilepsy patients: a 12-year observation. Neurology 2004;63:1124–6.

37. Revesz D, Tjernstrom M, Ben-Menachem E, et al. Effects of vagus nerve stimulation on rat hippocampal progenitor proliferation. Exp Neurol 2008; 214:259–65.

38. Cook IA, DeGiorgio CM, Miller PM, et al. Noninvasive neuromodulation with trigeminal nerve stimulation: a novel treatment for major depressive disorder. Poster presented at the NCDEU Annual Meeting. Boca Raton (FL), June 14–17, 2010.

Thalamic Stimulation for Epilepsy

Yinn Cher Ooi, BS[a], John C. Styliaras, MD[b],
Ashwini Sharan, MD[b],*

KEYWORDS

- Epilepsy • Seizures • Deep brain stimulation • Thalamus
- Anterior nucleus • Centromedian nucleus

Approximately one-third of patients with epilepsies experience persistent seizures despite maximal antiepileptic drug (AED) therapy.[1–3] Patients with refractory partial seizures may benefit from surgery, which may provide up to 90% reduction in seizure frequencies.[4] The surgical options used for medically refractory epilepsy include (1) lesionectomy: both temporal and extratemporal excisions of seizure focus; (2) lesionectomy with corticectomy: removing both the epileptogenic lesion with the surrounding cortex; (3) disconnection surgery: subpial transections to isolate the seizure focus from the rest of the brain, including corpus callosotomies, and (4) vagus nerve stimulation.[5–8] However, up to 50% of patients with medically intractable seizures either elect against these resective procedures or are deemed unsuitable candidates.[4]

With the growing number of applications for deep brain stimulation (DBS) in recent years, interest in using it as an option for patients with epilepsy has increased.[9,10] No consensus exists on the exact target for DBS for epilepsy, and therefore many sites are actively being explored. Candidates include the anterior nucleus of the thalamus (ANT), the centromedian nucleus of the thalamus (CMT), the subthalamic nucleus, and the hippocampus.

Even though the efficacy of DBS is becoming more evident, the exact mechanism through which DBS reduces seizure frequency is not fully understood. In patients with epilepsy, the brain oscillates between a functionally normal state and an abnormal ictal one, implying that the brain in patients with epilepsy is bistable or multistable.[11] DBS for epilepsy generally involves the chronic delivery of high-frequency stimulation, which has been hypothesized to establish or reinforce the functionally normal brain state and block epileptiform activity in the cortex.[12–15] In hippocampal slice model systems, high-frequency stimulation causes increased extracellular potassium accumulation and negative slow potential shifts, resulting in decreased neuronal excitability, and thus suppression of seizures.[16,17]

The target with the most promise seems to be located within the thalamus. Thalamic DBS has been reported for partial-onset epilepsy with or without secondary generalizations refractory to at least 12 to 18 months of two or more therapeutically dosed AEDs.[18–21] The benefit of DBS is usually palliative, although certain studies have reported patients to be complete seizure-free post-DBS.[22]

RATIONALE FOR STIMULATION OF THE ANT

The ANT is a crucial structure in the propagation of limbic epilepsy. In 1937, James W. Papez[23] described for the first time the circuit linking the

Drs. Ooi and Styliaras have nothing to disclose.
Dr Sharan's disclosures include: St. Jude: Grant support, Honorarium, Consultant fee; Medtronic: Honorarium, Consultant fee; Covidian: Consultant fee; Integra: Honorarium; IntElect: Stock/Shareholder; ICVRX: Founder, Consultant, Shareholder; NonLinear Technologies: Consultant; Zimmer Spine: Financial/medical support.
No funding support was received for the authorship of this article.
a Jefferson Medical College, Thomas Jefferson University, 1020 Locust Street, Room #157, Philadelphia, PA 19107, USA
b Department of Neurosurgery, Thomas Jefferson University Hospital, 909 Walnut Street, 2nd Floor, Philadelphia, PA 19107, USA
* Corresponding author.
E-mail address: ashwini.sharan@jefferson.edu

hippocampal output via the fornix and mamillary nucleus in the posterior hypothalamus to the ANT. The ANT then projects to the cingulum bundle just deep to the cingulated gyrus, which travels around the wall of the lateral ventricle to the parahippocampal cortex. This structure then completes the circuit by returning to the hippocampus.[23] Atrophy or sclerotic changes of any of the structures within this circuit have been noted in known causes of epilepsy, such as mesial temporal sclerosis.[24] Hence, investigators have hypothesized that stimulating targets within this circuit may result in direct anterograde cortical stimulation and concurrent cessation of seizures.

The ANT thus became a natural choice in DBS for epilepsy, especially considering that the ANT was the target for stereotactic lesioning for seizure control for many years.[25] Anatomically, the ANT is also preferred because of its small size but multiple projections into the limbic structures (cingulated cortex, amygdala, hippocampus, orbitofrontal cortex, and caudate) allowing the stimulation of wide regions of the neocortex. Lastly, the ANT is easily accessible through the ventricle and is not as deep or close to the basal vasculature compared with alternative sites, such as the mamillary nuclei.[26]

EVIDENCE FOR EPILEPSY TREATMENT
Animal Models

The ANT has been extensively investigated in animal models of epilepsy and in human trials. Mirski and colleagues[27] showed in a rat model that high-frequency stimulation (100 Hz) of the ANT elevated the threshold for pentylenetetrazol-induced seizures. Inversely, low-frequency stimulation (8 Hz) had a converse effect and was even proconvulsant in the absence of pentylenetetrazol. Furthermore, Hamani and colleagues[28,29] were able to achieve similar results in a rat model with pilocarpine-induced seizures, and showed that 500 μA was the optimal stimulus setting for providing significantly increased latency to seizure onset and status epilepticus.[29] High-frequency stimulation of the ANT or unilateral lesioning of the ANT and blocked with bilateral high-frequency stimulation of the ANT has also been shown to reduce seizure severity and frequency in the kainic acid model.[30,31] The investigators hypothesized that these effects were secondary to a form of functional, if not structural, microthalamotomy caused by high-frequency ANT stimulation.

Human Trials

The effects of DBS on epilepsy in animal models did not take long to inspire the start of human trials. Upton and colleagues[32] first described improvement in seizure frequencies with chronic bilateral stimulation on the ANT in four of six patients, one of whom was completely seizure-free at follow-up. Again, this effect could have been secondary to a form of functional microthalamotomy of the ANT. In a case series of five patients, Hodaie and colleagues[18] also reported a mean reduction in seizure frequency of greater than 50% after high-frequency stimulation of the ANT. The observed benefits did not differ between stimulation-on and stimulation-off periods. Subsequent studies have shown that electrode implantation itself decreases seizure frequencies (possibly from thalamotomy effect from insertion), and that activation of the implantable pulse generator (IPG) and multiple subsequent adjustments to stimulation parameters may not be directly linked to any further benefit in seizure control.[20,33] Andrade and colleagues[33] found that ANT DBS electrode implantation in six patients was followed by seizure reduction 1 to 3 months before active stimulation, again raising the possibility of a microthalamotomy effect.[33] Continued improved seizure control in a patient for more than a year after the pulse generators were turned off further suggests the primary role for the microthalamotomy in seizure control. However, Osorio and colleagues[21] were unable to detect any lesion effect with electrode insertion during the immediate postoperative period.

In a pilot study by Kerrigan and colleagues,[19] four of five patients who received intermittent ANT stimulation had a statistically significant reduction in frequency of secondarily generalized tonic-clonic seizures and complex partial seizures associated with falls. One patient showed a statistically significant reduction in total seizure frequency with active stimulation, and discontinuation of DBS stimulation resulted in an immediate increase in seizure frequency and vice versa. These findings also suggested the role of ANT stimulation in the reducing seizure frequency.[19-21]

Other studies improved on the statistical power of the initial small studies through recruiting multiple health care centers. In a large phase III multicenter trial, the Stimulation of the Anterior Nucleus of the Thalamus for Epilepsy trial (SANTE trial) sponsored by Medtronic (Minneapolis, MN, USA), patients were observed to have a reduction in seizure frequency after ANT DBS implantation and before active stimulation, indicating the presence of microthalamotomy effect.[22] However, a statistically significant reduction in seizure frequency in the stimulation group compared with the control group continued during the blinded phase of the study. Furthermore, continued reduction in seizure frequency occurred over time during long-term follow-up, and improvement in seizure control within the control group was also seen 4 months after initiation of stimulation. These findings clearly suggest an effect of stimulation independent of the microlesion effect of electrode implantation.[22]

During the blinded phase of the study, seizure frequency reduction was significantly greater in the stimulation group (38% reduction) versus the control group (15% reduction).[22] During long-term follow-up and open-label phase of the study, seizure frequency reduction as a function of stimulation was −40% at 13 months, −57% at 25 months, and −67% at 37 months.[22] The 50% responder rate was 41% at 13 months, 54% at 2 years, and 65% at 3 years.[22] Seizure freedom was observed for at least 6 months in 13 patients.[22] In addition, these improvements were seen in some participants who had not previously received multiple AEDs, vagus nerve stimulation, or epilepsy surgery.[22] The SANTE trial also reported an overall improvement of quality of life based on Quality-of-Life-in-Epilepsy (QoLIE-31) scores in the stimulation group.[18] The trial reported an outlier who had 210 seizures corresponding to the 5-minute stimulation cycle when the stimulator was turned on throughout the entire blinded phase of the study.[22] The stimulator was turned off and the new seizures stopped immediately. Subsequently, this patient improved as stimulator parameters were adjusted.

Seizure Type Localization

The localization of seizure focus may also affect the efficacy of ANT stimulation for seizure control. Bitemporal mesial epilepsy in comparison with extratemporal or poorly localized seizures confers different benefits of DBS.[18,19,33] Bitemporal mesial seizures seem to be more responsive to ANT stimulation than nonmesial ones. Osorio and colleagues[21] reported up to a 75% reduction in seizure frequency, and even a 93% reduction in seizure frequency in one patient with this type of epilepsy. However, in Osorio's study, a higher frequency of up to 157 Hz was used, which may partially explain the improved seizure response.

The SANTE trial also reported that the efficacy of ANT stimulation for seizure control depended on the region of seizure origin.[22] A statistically significant benefit in reduction of seizure frequency was reported in patients with seizure origin in one or both temporal regions, with a 44.2% reduction in seizure frequency within the stimulated group versus 21.8% in the control group ($P = .025$). Of these patients, 6% had a 100% reduction and approximately 19% had a 90% decrease in

seizure frequency. However, among patients with seizure origin within the frontal, parietal, or occipital regions no significant differences in seizure reduction were seen between the stimulated and control groups. The trial also reported a reduction in seizure frequency in patients with multifocal or diffuse seizures, with a 35% reduction in the stimulation group versus 14.1% in the control group. However, because of the small number of patients, the difference was not statistically significant.

TARGETING AND SURGICAL STEPS

The stereotactic head frame should be placed while the patient is under either local anesthesia or general endotracheal anesthesia.[18–21,33,34] The frame should be placed with a tilt parallel to the lateral canthus (the external auditory meatal line that is approximately parallel to the anterior commissure) and the posterior commissure line (AC-PC). Standard T2 and fast spine echo inversion recovery images should be obtained with a 1.5- or 3.0-Tesla MRI. Target site selection is obtained using 1-mm thick axial, coronal, and sagittal spoiled gradient echo pulse sequences. However a CT scan is also a viable alternative.

The ANT is localized indirectly with reference to the standard stereotactic atlas[35] through first indentifying the AC-PC line on the sagittal image. AC and PC coordinates relative to the center of the frame are obtained to calculate the midcommissural point (MCP). The ANT is 12 mm superior and 5 mm lateral to the MCP. Alternatively, the ANT can also be localized through direct visualization at the floor of the lateral ventricle on MRI, and the frame coordinates can be calculated. The entry point for lead insertion should be at or just anterior to the coronal suture. The simulated trajectory from the entry point is planned to ensure avoidance of sulcal vessels using a surgical navigation system. More frequently a target traversing the ventricle is used.

The patient should be placed either in a supine position or semisitting position. Either local or general anesthesia is acceptable. Bilateral burr holes are placed over the entry point. The dura and pia are incised sharply and cauterized. A guide cannula is inserted through the burrhole and advanced deep into the brain up to 10 mm from the desired target with direct fluoroscopic guidance. A monopolar single-unit recording electrode can be introduced to confirm anatomic depth and entry into thalamic tissue after traversing the lateral ventricle, however this is not essential. The first recordings indicate electrode tip entry into the ANT superficial surface with subsequent cessation in recordings indicating the intralaminar region and recommencement of recordings indicate tip entry into the dorsomedian nucleus of the thalamus. ANT neurons are identified based on (1) regional characteristics, (2) a firing rate previously described for human recordings,[19] and (3) a characteristic burst firing pattern.

The DBS lead is advanced to the ANT ensuring that all lead contacts are within the thalamic parenchyma. Frequently contacts will be placed beyond the ANT. The cannula and lead stylet are withdrawn under fluoroscopy and another fluoroscopic image is then taken to confirm that the electrode is secure. A burrhole cap is used to secure the lead, and the skin incision is closed.

The stereotactic head frame is removed and the head, neck, and subclavicular region are prepped sterile for implantation of the IPG (model Itrel II, Soletra, or Kinetra; Medtronic) in a subclavicular pocket bilaterally. The scalp incision is reopened to connect the stimulation leads to the extension wire (Medtronic 7495 Lead Extension; Medtronic), which is tunneled subcutaneously along the lateral aspect of the neck toward the subclavicular pocket and connected to the IPG. Before closure, the lead, extension, and IPG connection should be confirmed, with impedance checking performed through the IPG.

For DBS in the anterior nucleus of the thalamus, it is particularly important to obtain postoperative MR imaging to confirm positioning of the electrodes. Unlike with Parkinson disease, for which an implanter has both an obvious clinical response regarding a patient's rigidity and tremor and the ability to perform microelectrode recording, assessment and response of epilepsy may take time to maximize. Therefore, patients must receive the maximum opportunity to become a responder, which obviously includes placement of the electrode at the correct intended target.

STIMULATION SETTINGS

Stimulation settings are variable and can range between 90 and 130 Hz, a pulse width of 60 and 90 μs and an amplitude of 4 to 5 V using the contact that induces the optimal clinical effects at minimal voltage with the fewest side effects. Bipolar settings are preferred based on the assumption that the current generated should be more localized than unipolar.[20] However the benefits of bipolar stimulation over unipolar stimulation remain largely unknown. Additionally, a study by Lim and colleagues[20] reported no significant difference in seizure frequency control between cyclic and continuous stimulation in four patients with bilateral ANT DBS. Cyclic or intermittent stimulation improves battery life.[18] Cyclic stimulation is also theoretically safer for neural tissue than

chronic continuous stimulation.[18] Litt[9] proposed using an open-loop device for intermittent stimulation through a duty cycle of 1 minute on and 5 minutes off. The SANTE trial, which showed the efficacy of ANT DBS for seizure frequency control, adopted an initial stimulation setting of 145 Hz with a pulse amplitude of 5 V and a pulse width of 90 μs, using a cycle of 1 minute on and 5 minutes off stimulation.[22]

COMPLICATIONS

ANT stimulation seems to be a safe and well-tolerated procedure, with very minimal, mild, and transient complications associated with the procedure or stimulation. Numerous pilot studies involving human trials reported no adverse events attributed to ANT stimulation.[19,36] Reported complications associated with intermittent ANT stimulation include intermittent nystagmus, paranoid ideation, hallucinations, anorexia, and lethargy.[21,33,34] In the recent multicenter SANTE trial involving 110 patients, 2 experienced acute, transient, stimulus-linked seizures on stimulus initiation, both resolving with lowering voltage.[22] Although neuropsychological test scores for cognition and mood did not differ between control and stimulated groups at the end of the blinded phase, the investigators reported that stimulation may induce or worsen depression in certain patients, as observed in 8 patients within the study.

Complications secondary to the surgical procedure are similar to those previously described for DBS, and include scalp erosion and hardware exposure necessitating removal of the system; infection at the generator implant site; and hemorrhage.[18,20,37] The SANTE trial reported paresthesias (18.2%), implant site pain (10.9%), and implant site infection (9.1%) as the most common device-related adverse events.[22] No symptomatic or clinically significant hemorrhages occurred; however, neuroimaging showed that five patients (4.5%) had incidental hemorrhage.[22] Leads were initially implanted outside the ANT in nine patients (8.2%), and were subsequently replaced. (**Fig. 1**) The SANTE trial also reported two deaths attributed to sudden unknown death in epilepsy, one occurring during the unblinded phase and the other during the long-term follow-up phase. This rate of 6.2 per 1000 years is within expected range for the study population.[38]

CMT

Another target of DBS for medically intractable seizures is the CMT. In 1938, Penfield[39] first described the CMT as an integral part of the

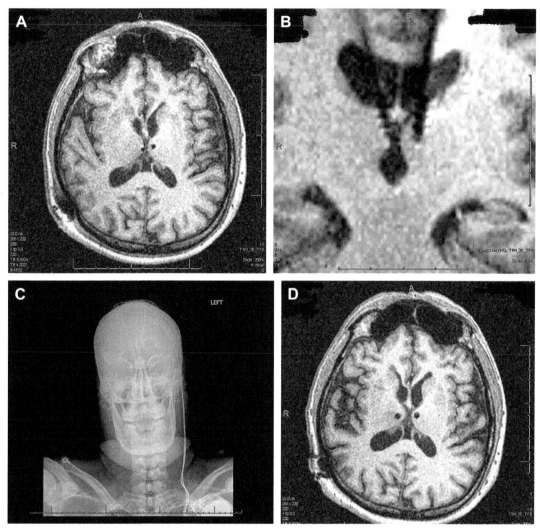

Fig. 1. Postoperative imaging was routinely performed after electrode implantation. (*A, B*) MR images showing medial positioning of the right DBS electrode. (*C*) represents an anteroposterior skull radiograph showing the same. The electrode on the right side was independently viewed by a neuroradiologist and the surgeon; both believed that the medial-most inferior contact may be in the ventricle. They recommended that the right electrode be revised. (*D*) shows the final position after revision of the right-sided DBS lead.

ascending subcortical system, arising from the brain stem and diencephalon and projecting diffusely to the cerebral cortex. This description provided the basis for implicating the role of CMT in the pathophysiology of generalized seizures. In 1984, Velasco and colleagues[39] began their work on addressing CMT DBS through implanting a bilateral CMT DBS in a 12-year-old with Lennox-Gastaut syndrome (LGS). Much of this work was derived from prior reports on electrical stimulation of the nonspecific thalamic nuclei by Morrison and Dempsey.[40] Velasco and colleagues[41] reported up to an 80% reduction in overall seizures and improvement in quality of life in 13 patients with LGS. However, the response

rate for patients with epilepsy who did not have LGS was less significant.[42] Stimulation did, however, seem to impede secondary generalization of patients with epilepsy who did not have LGS.[42] Velasco and colleagues[41,43] reported an 87% reduction in seizure frequency in patients with CMT stimulation with an average of 46 months of follow-up. Stimulation settings were maintained at 130 Hz, 0.45 ms, and 400 to 600 mA alternating in left/right 1-minute trains with a 4-minute quiescent interval phase.

Although CMT may seem to be effective in controlling frequency of generalized seizures, its usefulness in controlling the frequency of complex partial seizures remains largely unknown.[44–47]

Furthermore, in contrast to the open-label trials that showed the efficacy of CMT DBS in seizure control, double-blind studies report a lack of a statistically significant difference in seizure frequency and of short-term benefit.[33,48]

SUMMARY

Thalamic DBS, specifically ANT DBS, seems to be a viable minimally invasive treatment alternative for patients experiencing medically intractable seizures. Thalamic DBS has been associated with not only a significant reduction in seizure frequency but also an improvement in overall quality of life, especially in patients for whom maximal AEDs or other surgical alternatives have failed. Patients with seizure focus localized at the temporal lobes seem to experience the greatest benefit from ANT DBS. Recent evidence suggests that ANT DBS is a safe and well-tolerated procedure, with minimal, mild transient adverse effects associated with stimulation and implantation.

Further work is necessary to identify additional subgroups of patients experiencing medically intractable seizures who may benefit from ANT DBS, and further investigations are necessary to indentify optimal stimulation parameters and mode of stimulation.

SOCIAL IMPACT

In a personal correspondence, Fisher pointed out that based on the SANTE trial, if patients were assumed to have an average of 20 seizures a month and a conservative estimate of 100 new patients were implanted with ANT DBS each year, who would then show a 40% seizure reduction, a 5-year delay would lead to 48,000 additional seizures, including numerous associated injuries (Fisher R, personal communication, 2010). Certainly this would be a strong indication for using ANT DBS to treat epilepsy.

Europe's CE-Mark, involving 27 countries, has currently approved DBS for epilepsy based on the SANTE trial data and other accumulated experience in Europe and elsewhere.[49] Although a U.S. Food and Drug Administration (FDA) advisory panel recommended approval, the FDA indicated that approval in the United States will require more data to better establish the risk/benefit ratio.[50]

REFERENCES

1. Juul-Jensen P. Epidemiology of intractable epilepsy. In: Schmidt D, Morselli P, editors. Intractable epilepsy. New York: Raven Press; 1986. p. 5–11.
2. Sander JW. Some aspects of prognosis in the epilepsies: a review. Epilepsia 1993;34(6):1007–16.
3. Sillanpaa M, Schmidt D. Natural history of treated childhood-onset epilepsy: prospective, long-term population based study. Brain 2006;129(Pt 3): 617–24.
4. ILAE Commission Report. A global survey on epilepsy surgery, 1980–1990: a report by the Commission on Neurosurgery of Epilepsy, the International League Against Epilepsy. Epilepsia 1997; 38(2):249–55.
5. Cascino GD, Kelly PJ, Sharbrough FW, et al. Long term follow-up of stereotactic lesionectomy in partial epilepsy: predictive factors and electroencephalographic results. Epilepsia 1992;33:639–44.
6. Weber JP, Silbergeld DL, Winn HR. Surgical resection of epileptogenic cortex associated with structural lesions. Neurosurg Clin N Am 1993;4:327–36.
7. Smith MC. Multiple subpial transection in patients with extratemporal epilepsy. Epilepsia 1998; 39(Suppl 4):S81–9.
8. Spencer SS. Corpus callosum section and other disconnection procedures for medically intractable epilepsy. Epilepsia 1988;29(Suppl 2):S85–99.
9. Litt B. Evaluating devices for treating epilepsy. Epilepsia 2003;44(Suppl 7):30–7.
10. Litt B, Baltuch G. Brain stimulation for epilepsy. Epilepsy Behav 2001;2:S61–7.
11. Lopes da Silva F, Blanes W, Kalitzin SN, et al. Epilepsies as dynamical diseases of brain systems: basic models of the transition between normal and epileptic activity. Epilepsia 2003;44(Suppl 12):72–83.
12. Nagel SJ, Najm IM. Deep brain stimulation for epilepsy. Neuromodulation Technology at the Neural Interface 2009;12:270–80.
13. Monnier M, Kalberer M, Krupp P. Functional antagonism between diffuse reticular and intralaminar recruiting projections in the medial thalamus. Exp Neurol 1960;2:271–89.
14. Velasco M, Velasco F. State related brain stem regulation on cortical and motor excitability: effects on experimental focal motor seizures. Orlando (FL): Academic Press; 1982.
15. Lado FA, Velisek L, Moshe SL. The effect of electrical stimulation of the subthalamic nucleus on seizures is frequency dependent. Epilepsia 2003; 44(2):157–64.
16. Durand D. Electrical stimulation can inhibit synchronized neuronal activity. Brain Res 1986;382:139–44.
17. Gluckman BJ, Neel EJ, Netoff TI, et al. Electric field suppression of epileptiform activity in hippocampal slices. J Neurophysiol 1996;76:4202–5.
18. Hodaie M, Wennberg RA, Dostrovsky JO, et al. Chronic anterior thalamus stimulation for intractable epilepsy. Epilepsia 2002;43(6):603–8.
19. Kerrigan JF, Litt B, Fisher RS, et al. Electrical stimulation of the anterior nucleus of the thalamus for the treatment of intractable epilepsy. Epilepsia 2004; 45(4):346–54.

20. Lim SN, Lee ST, Tsai YT, et al. Electrical stimulation of the anterior nucleus of the thalamus for intractable epilepsy: a long-term follow-up study. Epilepsia 2007;48(2):342–7.

21. Osorio I, Overman J, Giftakis J, et al. High frequency thalamic stimulation for inoperable mesial temporal epilepsy. Epilepsia 2007;48(8):1561–71.

22. Fisher R, Salanova V, Witt T, et al. Electrical stimulation of the anterior nucleus of thalamus for treatment of refractory epilepsy. Epilepsia 2010;51(5):899–908.

23. Carpenter MB. Core text of neuroanatomy. 4th edition. Baltimore (MD): Williams & Wilkins; 1991.

24. Oikawa H, Sasaki M, Tamakawa Y, et al. The circuit of Papez in mesial temporal sclerosis: MRI. Neuroradiology 2001;43(3):205–10.

25. Mullan S, Vailati G, Karasick J, et al. Thalamic lesions for the control of epilepsy. A study of nine cases. Arch Neurol 1967;16(3):277–85.

26. Krames ES, Peckham PH, Rezai AR. Neuromodulation. London (UK), Burlington (MA), San Diego (CA): Sabre Foundation, Elsevier; 2009.

27. Mirski MA, Rossell LA, Terry JB, et al. Anticonvulsant effect of anterior thalamic high frequency electrical stimulation in the rat. Epilepsy Res 1997;28:89–100.

28. Hamani C, Ewerton FI, Bonilha SM, et al. Bilateral anterior thalamic nucleus lesions and high-frequency stimulation are protective against pilocarpine-induced seizures and status epilepticus. Neurosurgery 2004;54:191–7.

29. Hamani C, Hodaie M, Chiang J, et al. Deep brain stimulation of the anterior nucleus of the thalamus: effects of electrical stimulation on pilocarpine-induced seizures and status epilepticus. Epilepsy Res 2008;78:117–23.

30. Takebayashi S, Hashizume K, Tanaka T, et al. The effect of electrical stimulation and lesioning of the anterior thalamic nucleus on kainic acid-induced focal cortical seizure status in rats. Epilepsia 2007; 48:348–58.

31. Takebayashi S, Hashizume K, Tanaka T, et al. Anti-convulsant effect of electrical stimulation and lesioning of the anterior thalamic nucleus on kainic acid-induced focal limbic seizure in rats. Epilepsy Res 2007;74:163–70.

32. Upton AR, Cooper IS, Springman M, et al. Suppression of seizures and psychosis of limbic system origin by chronic stimulation of anterior nucleus of the thalamus. Int J Neurol 1985;19–20:223–30.

33. Andrade DM, Zumsteg D, Hamani C, et al. Long-term follow-up of patients with thalamic deep brain stimulation for epilepsy. Neurology 2006;66(10): 1571–3.

34. Samadani U, Baltuch GH. Anterior thalamic nucleus stimulation for epilepsy. Acta Neurochir 2007; 97(Suppl):1–4.

35. Schaltenbrand G, Wahren W. Atlas for Stereotaxy of the human brain. Stuttgart (Germany): Thieme; 1977.

36. Benabid AL, Minotti L, Koudsie A, et al. Antiepileptic effect of high-frequency stimulation of the subthalamic nucleus (corpus luysi) in a case of medically intractable epilepsy caused by focal dysplasia: a 30-month follow-up: technical case report. Neurosurgery 2002;50:1385–92.

37. Lee KJ, Jang KS, Shon YM. Chronic deep brain stimulation of subthalamic and anterior thalamic nuclei for controlling refractory partial epilepsy. Acta Neurochir Suppl 2006;99:87–91.

38. Dasheiff RM. Sudden unexpected death in epilepsy: a series from an epilepsy surgery program and speculation on the relationship to sudden cardiac death. J Clin Neurophysiol 1991;8(2):216–22.

39. Velasco M, Velasco F, Velasco AL, et al. Acute and chronic electrical stimulation of the centromedian thalamic VI. Neurostimulation for Epilepsy nucleus: modulation of reticulo-cortical systems and predictor factors for generalized seizure control. Arch Med Res 2000;31(3):304–15.

40. Morrison RS, Dempsey EW. A study of thalamocortical relations. Am J Physiol 1942;135:281–92.

41. Velasco AL, Velasco F, Jimenez F, et al. Neuromodulation of the centromedian thalamic nuclei in the treatment of generalized seizures and the improvement of the quality of life in patients with Lennox–Gastaut syndrome. Epilepsia 2006;47(7):1203–12.

42. Velasco F, Velasco AL, Velasco M, et al. Deep brain stimulation for treatment of the epilepsies: the centromedian thalamic target. Acta Neurochir Suppl 2007;97:337–42.

43. Velasco M, Velasco F, Velasco AL. Centromedian-thalamic and hippocampal electrical stimulation for the control of intractable epileptic seizures. J Clin Neurophysiol 2001;18:495–513.

44. Velasco M, Velasco F, Velasco AL, et al. Effect of chronic electrical stimulation of the centromedian thalamic nuclei on various intractable seizure patterns: II. Psychological performance and background EEG activity. Epilepsia 1993;34(6):1065–74.

45. Velasco F, Velasco M, Jimenez F, et al. Stimulation of the central median thalamic nucleus for epilepsy. Stereotact Funct Neurosurg 2001;77(1–4):228–32.

46. Velasco F, Velasco M, Ogarrio C, et al. Electrical stimulation of the centromedian thalamic nucleus in the treatment of convulsive seizures: a preliminary report. Epilepsia 1987;28(4):421–30.

47. Velasco F, Velasco M, Velasco AL, et al. Electrical stimulation of the centromedian thalamic nucleus in control of seizures: long-term studies. Epilepsia 1995;36(1):63–71.

48. Fisher RS, Uematsu S, Krauss GL, et al. Placebo-controlled pilot study of centromedian thalamic stimulation in treatment of intractable seizures. Epilepsia 1992;33(5):841–51.

49. Medtronic Receives European CE Mark Approval for Deep Brain Stimulation Therapy for Refractory

Epilepsy Further Clinical Study Required for Application to U.S. Food and Drug Administration. Medtronic Newsroom. Available at: http://wwwp.medtronic.com/Newsroom/NewsReleaseDetails.do?itemId51284644553533&lang5en_US. Accessed August 13, 2011.

50. Neurological Devices Panel of the Medical Devices Meeting Announcement. U.S. Food and Drug Administration. Available at: http://www.fda.gov/AdvisoryCommittees/Calendar/ucm199499.htm. Accessed August 13, 2011.

Hippocampal Stimulation in the Treatment of Epilepsy

Jose F. Tellez-Zenteno, MD, PhD[a], Samuel Wiebe, MD[b],*

KEYWORDS

• Deep brain stimulation • Epilepsy • Surgery • Hippocampus

Neuromodulation is one of the fastest growing fields in neurosurgery, as reflected by the growing interest in the use of electrical brain stimulation (EBS) to treat drug-resistant epilepsy, pain, and movement disorders. The use of EBS to treat neurologic symptoms began to flourish during the 1970s when totally subcutaneous implantable stimulation systems became available.[1] In the 1970s, Richardson and Akil[2,3] pioneered EBS of the periventricular and periaqueductal gray matter for the relief of peripheral and central pain, and Hosobuchi[4] used chronic EBS of the thalamus and internal capsule to treat central pain.

Cooper and colleagues[5] first showed a potential benefit of EBS in epilepsy in patients treated for seizures and for spasticity. In his initial study, published in 1973, 15 patients had EBS of the cerebellum and all had some level of improvement in frequency and severity of seizures. Cerebellar biopsies, obtained in 5 patients at the time of stimulator placement, revealed in every instance a reduction in the molecular layer, decreased or absent Purkinje cells, and decreased stellate cells. Cooper[6] claimed that EBS was safe because histologic examination of the brain did not reveal tissue damage attributable to the stimulator. In a subsequent study, Cooper and Upton[7] showed that 68 of 100 patients with cerebral palsy showed clinical improvement after chronic cerebellar EBS. Electroencephalographic studies done in some of the patients with epilepsy revealed a significant reduction of paroxysmal electroencephalogram (EEG) discharges during the stimulation and rebound increases after cessation of the stimulation.

After the pioneering work of Cooper and colleagues, Velasco and colleagues[8] explored the effect on seizures of centromedian-thalamic nucleus stimulation. In his initial study, he described the effect of EBS in 5 patients with generalized or focal drug-resistant seizures. All patients underwent stereotactic implantation of electrodes in both centromedian (CM) thalamic nuclei. Clinical seizures and EEG epileptiform discharges were significantly reduced by EBS. Subsequent studies from the same group showed similar results.[9,10]

Recently, a multicenter randomized blinded study explored the effect of EBS of the anterior nuclei of the thalamus for localization-related epilepsy.[11] Half of 110 patients were randomized to receive stimulation and half received no stimulation during a 3-month blinded phase, followed by unblinded stimulation for all patients in the study. The mean seizure frequency decreased by 14.5% in the control group and by 40% in the stimulated group during the first 3 months (blinded phase) of the study. By 2 years, 54% of patients had a seizure reduction of at least 50%, and 14 patients were seizure free for at least 6 months.

This work was supported by the Hopewell Professorship of Clinical Neurosciences Research, Hotchkiss Brain Institute, University of Calgary.
The authors have nothing to disclose.
[a] Division of Neurology, Department of Medicine, University of Saskatchewan, Saskatoon, Saskatchewan, Canada
[b] Department of Clinical Neurosciences, University of Calgary, 1403-29 Street Northwest, Calgary, Alberta T3H 3J6, Canada
* Corresponding author.
E-mail address: swiebe@ucalgary.ca

Neurosurg Clin N Am 22 (2011) 465–475
doi:10.1016/j.nec.2011.07.008

Five deaths occurred in the study but were not related to the implantation or stimulation.

THE PROBLEM OF MESIAL TEMPORAL LOBE EPILEPSY

Despite an armamentarium of at least 20 different antiepileptic drugs (AEDs), approximately 30% of patients with epilepsy remain refractory to all forms of pharmacotherapy. One of the commonest forms of medically intractable epilepsy is mesial temporal lobe epilepsy (MTLE). Based on a randomized controlled trial by Wiebe and colleagues,[12] clinical practice guidelines were generated that recommend that these patients undergo evaluation for brain surgery, usually anteromesial temporal lobe resection.[13] Approximately 50% of medically refractory patients are potential candidates for epilepsy surgery and most have MTLE. Although MTLE surgery is effective and generally safe, it carries risks to memory and naming functions. The most recent evidence synthesis shows that, after left temporal lobe resection, 44% of patients exhibit reliable declines in verbal memory, and 34% decline in naming function.[14] Mood and psychiatric disorders can worsen in up to 18% of patients,[15] and serious neurologic sequelae occur in about 2% of patients.[13] Furthermore, the ability of resective surgery to render patients seizure free in MTLE, although impressive, has stayed at around 60% since the advent of magnetic resonance imaging (MRI) 2 decades ago. Surgical effectiveness has not improved with the development of newer technology. Therefore, there is a need to develop new therapies that improve current surgical outcomes, and avoid the risks of irreversible brain surgery. Perhaps the most important reason for developing nonresective therapies in pharmacoresistant MTLE is that there is a group of patients who could be excellent surgical candidates, but cannot be operated because of risks to their memory function. These patients show adequate memory function on the temporal lobe that is to be operated, but not on the temporal lobe on the nonoperated side. Surgery in these patients carries a significant risk of memory loss.[16] In summary, the clinical rationale for EBS in MTLE is based on 3 important factors. First, resective brain surgery is irreversible and can produce adverse effects in a small but important minority of patients. Second, a sizable proportion of patients with medically intractable MTLE who undergo resective surgery are not rendered seizure free, and a sizable minority cannot have surgery because resection may be unsafe. Third, if effective, EBS could be applied to a wider group of people with epilepsy that is currently intractable.

MECHANISMS OF EBS IN EPILEPSY

The exact mechanism of action of EBS in epilepsy is not known. However, current evidence supports a neuromodulatory effect on cortical excitability that disrupts seizure generation either directly, or indirectly through subcortical neuronal circuits.[17] At a mechanistic level, the antiseizure effect of EBS is supported by at least 19 in vitro and in vivo studies in epilepsy models using direct current (DC) or single pulse stimulation,[18–25] low-frequency stimulation,[26–30] and high-frequency stimulation.[29,31–36]

The hypothesis that hippocampal stimulation (HS) is effective in MTLE is supported by 11 in vitro studies exploring the effect of electrical stimulation on the hippocampus (10 in animals[18,19,21,22,24,28,31,32,37,38] and 1 in human hippocampal slices[37]). All studies showed suppression of spontaneous epileptiform discharges using various forms of electrical stimulation. In addition, 6 studies explored HS in vivo in rats. Four showed a delay in seizure occurrence or in development of kindling,[25,27,39,40] 1 showed decrease in afterdischarges,[41] and 1 showed a decrease in spontaneous epileptiform activity.[23]

Clinical Studies of HS in Epilepsy

At least a dozen clinical studies support the hypothesis that HS has an antiseizure effect on MTLE. Three studies described a decrease in interictal epileptiform discharges[42–44] in response to HS. Eight studies (n = 49) reported the effect of HS on seizures.[42,44–50] In 4 (n = 38), continuous or cyclic HS abolished seizures entirely in 14 patients and improved seizures by 50% or more in 16, without any adverse effects.[45,48–50] Two studies have reported on responsive HS in 3 patients (ie, seizure detection software triggers the delivery of HS). Seizures were aborted effectively in 1 patient,[46] and improved by 58% in another.[47] There was no effect in 1 patient with bilateral HS.[47] In most studies, HS was performed on a short-term basis (<1 month) during preoperative intracranial EEG assessment. Patients then underwent resective surgery. The resected tissue showed no evidence of electrical injury. One study blinded stimulation status for the first month only, and then applied stimulation to all patients and assessed outcomes at 18 months. They found greater than 95% seizure reduction in 5 patients with normal MRIs, whereas 4 patients with hippocampal sclerosis achieved only 50% to 70%

seizure reduction. There were no deleterious neuropsychological effects.[48]

Studies of HS for epilepsy vary substantially in surgical technique and stimulation parameters. Some studies insert a single 4-contact electrode along the hippocampal longitudinal axis through a parieto-occipital burr hole (**Fig. 1**). Others use 2 quadripolar electrodes, implanted through 2 occipital burr holes. One electrode is placed in the amygdala and the other in the anterior part of the hippocampus on each side (**Fig. 2**). The choice of contacts to stimulate also varies. Some studies stimulate all contacts in the electrodes, other choose specific electrodes based on a certain number of epileptiform discharges. Stimulation parameters vary from continuous to cycling, with various durations of On and Off periods. Most studies use 90-microsecond pulses in trains of 60 to 200 Hz, applied at constant current (5 mA) or constant voltage (1–10 V), or at subthreshold amplitudes for side effects (usually sensory or visual phenomena).

This article highlights specific HS studies in epilepsy, focusing on the main findings and commenting on some strengths and weaknesses of the studies.

The initial study exploring HS in patients with MTLE was performed by Velasco and colleagues[51] and included 10 patients who were implanted bilaterally and observed for 16 days before undergoing temporal lobectomy. In 7 patients (70%), there was complete cessation of complex partial and secondarily generalized tonic clonic seizures, and cessation of interictal spikes by the sixth day. Three patients had improvement in seizures and spikes. The most evident and fast antiepileptic responses were found in 5 patients whose stimulation contacts were located at either the pes hippocampus close to the amygdaloid nuclei or at the anterior parahippocampal gyrus close to the entorhinal cortex, or the anterior perforate space. Histopathologic analysis of the stimulated areas

revealed no changes related to the HS. Velasco and colleagues[51] concluded that HS is a safe and effective procedure. The proposed mechanism was the activation of the perforant pathway through a polysynaptic inhibitory influence on epileptogenic neurons in CA1 to CA4, and a change in benzodiazepine and opioid receptors produced by HS.

This initial study supporting the use of HS in patients with temporal lobe epilepsy showed that short-term HS is safe and exerted a remarkable beneficial effect on seizures. Weaknesses of the study include a small sample size, a short period of observation after implantation, and the lack of controls, randomization, or blinding.

The second study supporting the use of HS in temporal lobe epilepsy was performed by Vonck and colleagues.[50] This study analyzed 3 patients with normal MRI but electroclinical findings consistent with mesial temporal epilepsy. Two quadripolar deep brain stimulation electrodes were implanted in each hemisphere trough 2 occipital burr holes. All patients had unilateral stimulation of specific electrodes selected by a given number of epileptiform discharges. At 7 days of follow-up, 2 of the 3 patients had fewer seizures, and all had a reduction in the number of interictal spikes. After a mean follow-up of 5 months, all patients had a greater than 50% reduction in seizure frequency, and none experienced side effects. The investigators suggested that long-term HS in the ictal zone reduces spikes and seizures, but commented that implantation alone could produce improvement in seizure frequency.

This study showed a potential benefit and safety of hippocampal HS after a few months of treatment. Weaknesses include a small sample size, and the lack of controls, randomization, or blinding. Participants were selected from a large initial pool of patients with intractable temporal lobe epilepsy, suggesting that HS may be applicable only to a small, select group of patients.

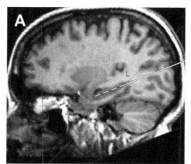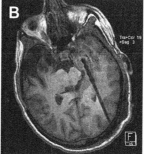

Fig. 1. T1-weighted MRI images showing HS surgical planning (*A*) and implantation (*B*), using a single quadripolar electrode along the longitudinal axis of the left hippocampus inserted through a parieto-occipital burr hole. L, left.

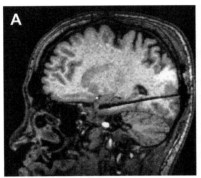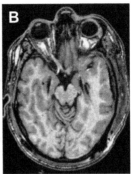

Fig. 2. MRI showing susceptibility artifacts of (*A*) left amygdalar electrode in a sagittal plane and (*B*) left amygdalar and hippocampal electrode and right amygdalar electrode in a coronal plane. (*Reproduced from* Boon P, Vonck K, De Herdt V, et al. Deep brain stimulation in patients with refractory temporal lobe epilepsy Epilepsia 2007;48(8):1551–60; with permission.)

The same group[45] studied 12 patients with refractory mesial temporal epilepsy who required intracranial EEG recording because of normal MRI or incongruent results of the noninvasive presurgical evaluation. Ten had seizure outcomes assessed at 12 to 52 months (mean 31 months). One of 10 patients had a greater than 90% reduction in seizure frequency, 5 had a seizure frequency reduction of 50% or more, 2 had a seizure frequency reduction of 30% to 49%, and 1 did not improve. One patient (8%) had asymptomatic hemorrhages along the trajectory of the depth electrodes. Two of the 12 patients with the poorest response to HS subsequently had resective surgery and were rendered seizure free. In most patients, the number of AEDs was lower at the end of follow-up. The investigators suggest that the mechanism of HS is related to the hypothesis of a reversible functional lesion. In this theory, local inhibition affects the areas that are involved in triggering, sustaining, and propagating epileptic activity.

As in the previous study by this group,[50] HS was safe and had a beneficial effect after few months of treatment. However, the study also indicates that observation of larger numbers of patients can identify complications that are not apparent with limited sample sizes. The weaknesses of the study include small sample size, and the lack of controls, randomization, and blinding. Two patients who initially were considered for HS eventually had a temporal lobectomy and were rendered seizure free.

Velasco and colleagues[48] performed a second study in 9 patients to evaluate the safety and efficacy of HS. All patients had intracranial EEG recordings because of potential bitemporal seizure onset. During the first month of the study, 5 patients were randomly assigned to the stimulator

being turned off, and 4 patients to the stimulator turned on. The stimulator was turned on in all patients after 1 month, and the main analysis was done at 18 to 84 months (average 37 months). Three patients had skin erosion and a local infection after 24 months' implantation. Five patients had normal MRIs and a seizure reduction of greater than 95%. Four patients had hippocampal sclerosis on MRI and their seizure reduction was only 50% to 70%. Neuropsychological testing before and after HS showed no changes. Patients randomized to 1-month stimulator turned on had both an immediate (1-month) and a late marked improvement in seizures, whereas those randomized to 1-month stimulator turned off had only late improvement in seizures and these were not as homogeneously favorable as those of the patients whose stimulator was on during the first month. The investigators concluded that HS is an alternative therapy for patients with mesial temporal epilepsy with normal MRI who are not candidates for epilepsy surgery.

There are several strong aspects of this study, including the longer follow-up, before-and-after neuropsychological assessment, and the analysis based on MRI findings. The brief, single randomized period and the small sample have negligible power and contribute little to the analysis. The investigators report that delaying stimulation by 1 month (stimulator off group) results in less favorable long-term seizure outcomes. This finding can hardly be attributed to the intervention and is more likely an artifact of the small sample size and perhaps inadequate long-term blinding. The investigators indicate that HS is useful where surgery is not indicated.

In a truly double-blind, randomized controlled trial, Tellez-Zenteno and colleagues[52] studied 4 patients with unilateral MTLE and hippocampal sclerosis who were not candidates for resective surgery because of substantial risk of memory loss. One quadripolar electrode was inserted along the longitudinal axis of the hippocampus through a parieto-occipital burr hole. A within-patient, double-blind, multiple crossover, randomized controlled design (N-of-1 randomized trial) was used, with paired randomization of On and Off treatment sequences in each patient. The On and Off treatment periods lasted 1 month each, and each patient completed 3 pairs of treatment periods (6 treatment periods of 1-month duration each). Outcomes were assessed at monthly intervals in a double-blind manner, using standardized instruments and accounting for a washout period. The comparison between On and Off periods showed a median percent reduction in seizure frequency of 15% during the On periods. Comparison with seizure frequency at baseline showed a median reduction of 26% when the stimulator was on, and an increase of 49% when the stimulator was off (**Fig. 3**). The absolute difference from baseline between On and Off groups was 75% favoring HS. One patient had no improvement in seizure frequency with HS. Neuropsychological function was comprehensively assessed at the end of each treatment period (6 times per patient), using alternate forms of the Boston Naming Test, Digit Span Test, Hopkins Verbal Learning Test, Brief Visual Memory Test, and Memory Assessment Clinic Self-Rating Scale. No differences were found between On and Off periods, or before and after HS in any of the tests. One patient who had a previous failed right temporal lobectomy improved dramatically with contralateral HS and showed no change in any of the cognitive tests. There were no differences

between On and Off periods in outcomes such as depression, quality of life, seizure severity, impact of epilepsy, and individual symptoms. The investigators concluded that the seizure control with HS was substantially more modest than in all previous studies, likely related to the true randomized, blinded nature of the study, compared with largely open-label, nonrandomized comparisons in other studies showing larger improvements. The short duration of treatment periods could also have contributed, and an implantation effect could not be excluded. A large-scale, double-blind, parallel-group, randomized controlled trial to adequately assess the effect of HS was recommended.

Although the sample size was small, the within-patient multiple randomized crossovers allowed for meaningful comparisons. The blinded, randomized comparison is the main strength of this study, including an analysis between On and Off periods. The 2 main weaknesses are the short treatment periods and the crossover design. HS periods of only 1 month may not be sufficient to obtain an effect. The crossover design is problematic because it is impossible to know with certainty whether the basic tenet to perform crossover studies is fulfilled in HS, that is, that all parameters return to baseline between treatment periods. There could be a cumulative effect of HS that continues after HS is turned off. This effect would decrease the difference between On and Off periods, spuriously decreasing the true effect of HS.

McLachlan conducted a blinded, single crossover, randomized trial in 2 patients using bitemporal HS.[25] The 2 patients were poor candidates for resective surgery because of the presence of independent bitemporal originating seizures. After

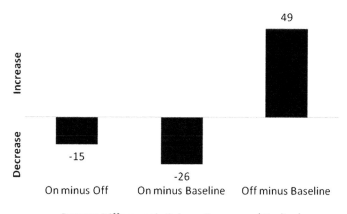

Fig. 3. Median percent change in seizure frequency in a multiple crossover, double-blind, randomized controlled trial by Tellez-Zenteno and colleagues.[52] The differences between On and Off periods were statistically significant.

a 3-month baseline period, patients were randomized to a 3-month period of HS on or off, followed by a 3-month washout period and a crossover 3 months to the opposite treatment (on or off). During the On period, the mean monthly seizure frequency decreased by 33% compared with the Off period. During the washout period, seizure frequency was still 25% lower despite no ongoing HS, suggesting an enduring effect of HS, and confirming that crossover designs are problematic in HS. Visuospatial memory during the On period worsened in 1 patient (decline from 21st to 1st percentile) and improved in the other (increase from 8th to 34th percentile), but there was substantial variation in this test during washout and Off study periods as well. Verbal and subjective memory did not change. No serious adverse effects were found in the 2 investigated patients. This study could not reproduce the impressive results reported by Velasco[51] and Vonck.[50] The patient with the better response had a normal MRI, suggesting that HS could be more useful in nonlesional patients, as suggested by Velasco.[51]

The study limitation of small sample size is self-evident. Strengths include the duration of the treatment period and the 3-month washout period, which suggests a persistent effect of HS, lasting several months after it is turned off. The study also suggests that implantation of the electrode itself did not decrease seizure frequency, which is important in the design of future studies (ie, On-Off comparisons are sufficient and no medical arm without implantation is needed). As in the study of Tellez-Zenteno and colleagues,[52] the seizure effect was less impressive than in unblinded, nonrandomized studies. The changes in neuropsychological function are of unknown relevance.

Ongoing Randomized Trials of HS

Two ongoing randomized controlled trials of HS are registered in Clinicaltrials.gov, the trials registry and results database of the National Institutes of Health.

One is a Canadian multicenter study led by Wiebe and colleagues, exploring the effect of HS on disabling seizures, with a secondary analysis of cognitive outcomes, quality of life, mood, and surgical complications. The design consists of a 3-month baseline period followed by a parallel-group, double-blind, randomized trial of on versus off HS for 7 months in patients with MTLE who may be candidates for resective surgery but whose memory function precludes surgery. The eligibility criteria for this study include patients with unilateral or bilateral mesial temporal epilepsy, 18 years of age or older, global intelligence

quotient (IQ) greater than 70, failure of adequate trials of 2 or more AEDs, ability to self-complete questionnaires, and patients' preference for nonresective surgery or not being a candidate for mesial temporal resection. The study is in progress and no results have been released.

The other ongoing study, led by Boon and colleagues in Belgium, is a single-blinded, parallel-group, 3-arm, randomized controlled trial comparing traditional anteromesial temporal resection, hippocampal electrode implantation with HS on, and hippocampal electrode implantation with HS off for the first 6 months. The primary outcome is mean seizure reduction, whereas secondary outcomes include neuropsychological function, quality of life, mood, and safety. Eligibility criteria include pharmacoresistant MTLE shown by video-EEG, age greater than 18 years, IQ greater than 80, ability to adequately report seizures, and MRI suggestive of hippocampal sclerosis.

In summary, the available evidence for HS is weak (**Table 1**). Many of the studies are small and of short duration, without controls or blinded outcome assessment. There seems to be a discrepancy in results from nonrandomized and randomized blinded studies, the latter showing significantly poorer effects of HS. The limited evidence suggests that the effects of HS seem to be cumulative and accrue with time, and the procedure seems to be safe. Neither the optimum target (amygdala, hippocampus, pes hippocampus, parahippocampal gyrus) nor the optimum stimulation parameters are known. However, variable improvement in seizures is reported in all studies of HS regardless of technique, and in virtually all studies of brain electrical stimulation for seizures. Subgroups of patients with MTLE who may benefit most from HS have not been identified, but there is a suggestion that patients with normal MRI may benefit more than those with mesial temporal sclerosis.

DISCUSSION

Like other forms of electrical neuromodulation, HS for mesial MTLE holds the promise of an intervention that is nonresective, minimally invasive, dose adjustable, largely reversible, and presumably safe. However, closer analysis of electrical stimulation of the brain for epilepsy reveals how little is known about this intervention, and how tenuous are the bases for this promise. For example, although the intervention is not evidently resective and it is clearly less invasive than standard resective surgery for epilepsy, detailed neuropsychological testing has not been done to assess the effects of implanting 1 or 2 electrodes along the longitudinal axis of the hippocampus, traversing the parieto-occipital cortex. The stimulation parameters are adjustable; however, optimum parameters are not known. It is remarkable that virtually all open-label electrical stimulation studies in epilepsy report beneficial effects, regardless of the stimulation target (thalamus, subthalamus, neocortex, hippocampus, cerebellum, and so forth), whether stimulation is administered at low or high frequency, continuously or intermittently, at rapid or slow cycles, at high or low amplitude, through monopolar or bipolar circuits, and using a few or all contacts in the electrode. The apparent ability of all modalities of electrical stimulation to improve seizures reflects either a remarkably robust class effect of the intervention, or remarkably poorly designed studies unable to yield a valid effect size. The reversibility of HS, supported partly by histopathologic integrity of the stimulated tissue and lack of overt clinical or EEG changes on short-term studies, is also alluring. However, almost nothing is known about the late or long-lasting effects of electrical stimulation on synaptic physiology, connectivity, function, and epileptogenicity. Studies with longer follow-up, such as the SANTE (Stimulation of the Anterior Nucleus of the Thalamus for Epilepsy) trial, suggest that electrical stimulation of the brain has a cumulative and variably enduring effect.[11] HS seems safe in the limited studies available. There is no convincing evidence on formal cognitive testing that HS produces consistent changes, whether patients undergo left, right, or bilateral HS. However, larger studies with longer follow-up, using other anatomic targets, have reported, for example, a higher incidence of depression with anterior thalamic stimulation. The long-term safety of HS is not known.

Reports of small, unblinded, nonrandomized HS studies of short duration have contributed to the enthusiasm for this intervention by showing significant or even dramatic seizure improvement. By contrast, preliminary studies of HS with more rigorous methods, including double blinding, randomized allocation of therapy, and blinded assessment of results, have yielded substantially and consistently less impressive results, which are more in line with those of the large randomized trial of anterior thalamic stimulation (SANTE trial).[11] In the SANTE trial, seizure freedom was rare in the blinded phase, and median seizure reduction was about 30% compared with no stimulation.

Researchers have heeded the call for scientifically robust evidence in HS, and have commenced blinded randomized controlled trials to establish an unbiased estimate of the effect size of HS on seizures, cognitive function, quality of life, mood, and surgical complications. However, these trials are difficult to perform and feasibility is continuously threatened. The reasons are many. First, surgical randomized trials are generally unpalatable to patients and clinicians. Second, the more rigorous studies suggest that electrical stimulation does not seem to have as dramatic an effect on seizures as traditional resective surgery, therefore clinicians are less motivated to refer patients for a trial of a potentially less effective intervention. Third, anteromesial temporal lobe resection is highly effective (number needed to treat of 2), the effects are durable and robust (results are similar in any region of the world), and it improves quality of life. The risks, in particular for memory and naming, are well known, and patients can be selected and counseled accordingly. Most patients with drug-resistant temporal lobe epilepsy are candidates for anteromesial resection, which leaves a small pool of patients to draw from for randomized trials of HS (eg, patients with a clear aversion to resective surgery, at high risk for cognitive decline, with bilaterally originating seizures, or those who failed temporal lobe resection and present with seizures in the contralateral mesial temporal structures). Fourth, funding for such trials is difficult to obtain, particularly because funding agencies ponder the risks of not enrolling sufficient patients and the existence of a highly effective surgical intervention for temporal lobe epilepsy. However, there is an urgent need for scientifically robust evidence about the effect HS on temporal lobe epilepsy, and about brain electrical stimulation for epilepsy in general. Whether HS is superior, inferior, or equivalent to resective surgery is unknown.

HS should be regarded as an experimental therapy for epilepsy, and patients should be considered for this intervention in the context of a well-designed, randomized controlled trial. At present, HS may be considered for patients with contraindication for a resective procedure because of risks to memory and naming functions or because of bitemporal epilepsy, as well as for patients with a strong stated preference for a nonresective, minimally invasive procedure. In the context of a well-designed randomized trial, HS might also be considered as an intermediate step before resective surgery, provided that availability of resources, waiting times for resective surgery, and ethical aspects are carefully accounted for. Only well-conducted, blinded, randomized trials, followed by long-term systematic observation, will yield a clear picture of the effect of this promising therapy, and will help guide its future use.

Table 1
Studies exploring hippocampal stimulation in MTLE

Study	Sample Size	Stimulation Parameters	Follow-up	Controlled Study/Randomization	Outcome	Study Limitations
Velasco et al,[51] 2000	10	Pulse width: 450 microseconds; Frequency: 130 Hz; Output: 200–400 mA (subthreshold); Electrodes: monopolar, all electrodes; Cycle: 23 h of every 24 h	16 d, before temporal lobectomy	None/none	In 70% of patients, seizure were abolished in the period of observation	Small sample size; short period of observation; lack of controls, randomization, or blinding
Vonck et al,[50] 2002	3	Pulse width: 450 microseconds; Frequency: 130–200 Hz; Patients 1 and 2 responded to the initial stimulation; Output: 1–3 V; Electrodes: bipolar, selected by number of spikes; Cycle: continuous	3–6 mo	None/none	Seizure reduction: 50% in all patients	Small sample size; lack of controls, randomization, and blinding
Boon et al,[45] 2007	12	Pulse width: 450 microseconds; Frequency: 130–200 Hz; Patients 1 and 2 responded to the initial stimulation; Output: 2–3 V; Electrodes: bipolar, selected by number of spikes; Cycle: continuous	12–52 mo, mean 31 mo	None/none	Seizure reduction: >90% in 1 patient; ≥50% in 5 patients; 30%–49% in 2 patients; 0% in 1 patient	Small sample size; lack of controls, randomization, and blinding

Study	N	Parameters	Duration	Design	Results	Limitations
Velasco et al,[48] 2007	9	Pulse width: 450 microseconds Frequency: 130 Hz Output: 200–400 mA (subthreshold) Electrodes: monopolar, all electrodes Cycle: intermittent 1 min On, 4 min Off	18–84 mo, mean 37 mo	Yes/yes On vs Off during first month of the study, then analyzed as single group	Seizure reduction: 95% if normal MRI 50%–70% if MTS on MRI	Small sample size, brief and single randomized period, which precludes strong conclusions
Tellez-Zenteno et al,[52] 2006	4	Pulse width: 90 microseconds Frequency: 190 Hz Output: 1.8–4.5 V (subthreshold) Electrodes: monopolar, all electrodes Cycle: continuous	6 mo	Yes/yes Double blind, On vs Off every month for 6 mo with multiple crossover trials in each patient	Seizure reduction: 15% On vs Off 26% On vs baseline Seizure increase: 49% Off vs baseline	Small sample size, short treatment periods, and crossover design
McLachlan, 2010	2	Pulse width: 90 microseconds Frequency: 185 Hz Output: 1.8–4.5 V (subthreshold) Electrodes: monopolar, all electrodes Cycle: continuous	9 mo	Yes/yes Double blind, On vs Off single crossover trial with washout period	Seizure reduction: 33% On vs Off 25% during washout	Small sample size

Abbreviation: MTS, mesial temporal sclerosis.

REFERENCES

1. Rise MT. Instrumentation for neuromodulation. Arch Med Res 2000;31(3):237–47.
2. Richardson DE, Akil H. Pain reduction by electrical brain stimulation in man. Part 1: acute administration in periaqueductal and periventricular sites. J Neurosurg 1977;47(2):178–83.
3. Richardson DE, Akil H. Pain reduction by electrical brain stimulation in man. Part 2: chronic self-administration in the periventricular gray matter. J Neurosurg 1977;47(2):184–94.
4. Hosobuchi Y, Adams JE, Rutkin B. Chronic thalamic and internal capsule stimulation for the control of central pain. Surg Neurol 1975;4(1):91–2.
5. Cooper IS, Amin I, Gilman S. The effect of chronic cerebellar stimulation upon epilepsy in man. Trans Am Neurol Assoc 1973;98:192–6.
6. Cooper IS, Amin I, Riklan M, et al. Chronic cerebellar stimulation in epilepsy. Clinical and anatomical studies. Arch Neurol 1976;33(8):559–70.
7. Cooper IS, Upton AR. Effects of cerebellar stimulation on epilepsy, the EEG and cerebral palsy in man. Electroencephalogr Clin Neurophysiol Suppl 1978;34:349–54.
8. Velasco F, Velasco M, Ogarrio C, et al. Electrical stimulation of the centromedian thalamic nucleus in the treatment of convulsive seizures: a preliminary report. Epilepsia 1987;28(4):421–30.
9. Velasco M, Velasco F, Velasco AL, et al. Acute and chronic electrical stimulation of the centromedian thalamic nucleus: modulation of reticulo-cortical systems and predictor factors for generalized seizure control. Arch Med Res 2000;31(3):304–15.
10. Velasco M, Velasco F, Velasco AL, et al. Effect of chronic electrical stimulation of the centromedian thalamic nuclei on various intractable seizure patterns: II. Psychological performance and background EEG activity. Epilepsia 1993;34(6):1065–74.
11. Fisher R, Salanova V, Witt T, et al. Electrical stimulation of the anterior nucleus of thalamus for treatment of refractory epilepsy. Epilepsia 2010;51(5):899–908.
12. Wiebe S, Blume WT, Girvin JP, et al. A randomized, controlled trial of surgery for temporal-lobe epilepsy. N Engl J Med 2001;345(5):311–8.
13. Engel J Jr, Wiebe S, French J, et al. Practice parameter: temporal lobe and localized neocortical resections for epilepsy: report of the Quality Standards Subcommittee of the American Academy of Neurology, in Association with the American Epilepsy Society and the American Association of Neurological Surgeons. Neurology 2003;60(4):538–47.
14. Sherman EM, Wiebe S, Fay-McClymont TB, et al. Neuropsychological outcomes after epilepsy surgery: systematic review and pooled estimates. Epilepsia 2011;52(5):857–69. DOI:10.1111/j.1528-1167.2011.03022.x.
15. Macrodimitris S, Sherman EM, Forde S, et al. Psychiatric outcomes of epilepsy surgery: a systematic review. Epilepsia 2011;52(5):880–90.
16. Kapur N, Prevett M. Unexpected amnesia: are there lessons to be learned from cases of amnesia following unilateral temporal lobe surgery? Brain 2003;126(Pt 12):2573–85.
17. Loddenkemper T, Pan A, Neme S, et al. Deep brain stimulation in epilepsy. J Clin Neurophysiol 2001;18(6):514–32.
18. Duong DH, Chang T. The influence of electric fields on the epileptiform bursts induced by high potassium in CA3 region of rat hippocampal slice. Neurol Res 1998;20(6):542–8.
19. Ghai RS, Bikson M, Durand DM. Effects of applied electric fields on low-calcium epileptiform activity in the CA1 region of rat hippocampal slices. J Neurophysiol 2000;84(1):274–80.
20. Gluckman BJ, Neel EJ, Netoff TI, et al. Electric field suppression of epileptiform activity in hippocampal slices. J Neurophysiol 1996;76(6):4202–5.
21. Kayyali H, Durand D. Effects of applied currents on epileptiform bursts in vitro. Exp Neurol 1991;113(2):249–54.
22. Nakagawa M, Durand D. Suppression of spontaneous epileptiform activity with applied currents. Brain Res 1991;567(2):241–7.
23. Richardson KA, Gluckman BJ, Weinstein SL, et al. In vivo modulation of hippocampal epileptiform activity with radial electric fields. Epilepsia 2003;44(6):768–77.
24. Warren RJ, Durand DM. Effects of applied currents on spontaneous epileptiform activity induced by low calcium in the rat hippocampus. Brain Res 1998;806(2):186–95.
25. McLachlan RS, Pigott S, Tellez-Zenteno JF, et al. Bilateral hippocampal stimulation for intractable temporal lobe epilepsy: impact on seizures and memory. Epilepsia 2010;51(2):304–7.
26. D'Arcangelo G, Panuccio G, Tancredi V, et al. Repetitive low-frequency stimulation reduces epileptiform synchronization in limbic neuronal networks. Neurobiol Dis 2005;19(1–2):119–28.
27. Goodman JH, Berger RE, Tcheng TK. Preemptive low-frequency stimulation decreases the incidence of amygdala-kindled seizures. Epilepsia 2005;46(1):1–7.
28. Khosravani H, Carlen PL, Velazquez JL. The control of seizure-like activity in the rat hippocampal slice. Biophys J 2003;84(1):687–95.
29. Mirski MA, Rossell LA, Terry JB, et al. Anticonvulsant effect of anterior thalamic high frequency electrical stimulation in the rat. Epilepsy Res 1997;28(2):89–100.
30. Psatta DM. Control of chronic experimental focal epilepsy by feedback caudatum stimulations. Epilepsia 1983;24(4):444–54.

31. Bikson M, Lian J, Hahn PJ, et al. Suppression of epileptiform activity by high frequency sinusoidal fields in rat hippocampal slices. J Physiol 2001; 531(Pt 1):181–91.

32. Lian J, Bikson M, Sciortino C, et al. Local suppression of epileptiform activity by electrical stimulation in rat hippocampus in vitro. J Physiol 2003; 547(Pt 2):427–34.

33. Morimoto K, Goddard GV. The substantia nigra is an important site for the containment of seizure generalization in the kindling model of epilepsy. Epilepsia 1987;28(1):1–10.

34. Nanobashvili Z, Chachua T, Nanobashvili A, et al. Suppression of limbic motor seizures by electrical stimulation in thalamic reticular nucleus. Exp Neurol 2003;181(2):224–30.

35. Velisek L, Veliskova J, Moshe SL. Electrical stimulation of substantia nigra pars reticulata is anticonvulsant in adult and young male rats. Exp Neurol 2002; 173(1):145–52.

36. Vercueil L, Benazzouz A, Deransart C, et al. High-frequency stimulation of the subthalamic nucleus suppresses absence seizures in the rat: comparison with neurotoxic lesions. Epilepsy Res 1998;31(1): 39–46.

37. Gluckman BJ, Nguyen H, Weinstein SL, et al. Adaptive electric field control of epileptic seizures. J Neurosci 2001;21(2):590–600.

38. Weiss SR, Li XL, Rosen JB, et al. Quenching: inhibition of development and expression of amygdala kindled seizures with low frequency stimulation. Neuroreport 1995;6(16):2171–6.

39. McIntyre DC, Poulter MO, Gilby K. Kindling: some old and some new. Epilepsy Res 2002;50(1–2): 79–92.

40. Velisek L, Veliskova J, Stanton PK. Low-frequency stimulation of the kindling focus delays basolateral amygdala kindling in immature rats. Neurosci Lett 2002;326(1):61–3.

41. Wyckhuys T, De ST, Claeys P, et al. High frequency deep brain stimulation in the hippocampus modifies seizure characteristics in kindled rats. Epilepsia 2007;48(8):1543–50.

42. Boex C, Vulliemoz S, Spinelli L, et al. High and low frequency electrical stimulation in non-lesional temporal lobe epilepsy. Seizure 2007;16(8):664–9.

43. Chkhenkeli SA, Sramka M, Lortkipanidze GS, et al. Electrophysiological effects and clinical results of direct brain stimulation for intractable epilepsy. Clin Neurol Neurosurg 2004;106(4):318–29.

44. Yamamoto J, Ikeda A, Satow T, et al. Low-frequency electric cortical stimulation has an inhibitory effect on epileptic focus in mesial temporal lobe epilepsy. Epilepsia 2002;43(5):491–5.

45. Boon P, Vonck K, De Herdt V, et al. Deep brain stimulation in patients with refractory temporal lobe epilepsy. Epilepsia 2007;48(8):1551–60.

46. Kossoff EH, Ritzl EK, Politsky JM, et al. Effect of an external responsive neurostimulator on seizures and electrographic discharges during subdural electrode monitoring. Epilepsia 2004;45(12):1560–7.

47. Osorio I, Frei MG, Sunderam S, et al. Automated seizure abatement in humans using electrical stimulation. Ann Neurol 2005;57(2):258–68.

48. Velasco AL, Velasco F, Velasco M, et al. Electrical stimulation of the hippocampal epileptic foci for seizure control: a double-blind, long-term follow-up study. Epilepsia 2007;48(10):1895–903.

49. Velasco AL, Velasco M, Velasco F, et al. Subacute and chronic electrical stimulation of the hippocampus on intractable temporal lobe seizures: preliminary report. Arch Med Res 2000;31(3):316–28.

50. Vonck K, Boon P, Achten E, et al. Long-term amygdalohippocampal stimulation for refractory temporal lobe epilepsy. Ann Neurol 2002;52(5):556–65.

51. Velasco M, Velasco F, Velasco AL, et al. Subacute electrical stimulation of the hippocampus blocks intractable temporal lobe seizures and paroxysmal EEG activities. Epilepsia 2000;41(2):158–69.

52. Tellez-Zenteno JF, McLachlan RS, Parrent A, et al. Hippocampal electrical stimulation in mesial temporal lobe epilepsy. Neurology 2006;66(10):1490–4.

Responsive Neurostimulation for the Treatment of Epilepsy

Paul R. Gigante, MD[a],*, Robert R. Goodman, MD, PhD[a,b]

KEYWORDS
• Epilepsy • Neurostimulation • Responsive • Seizures
• Neurostimulator

EARLY NEUROSTIMULATION IN EPILEPSY

The application of electrical stimulation as a means of modifying seizure activity has persisted since the development of early experimental epilepsy models and intraoperative seizure focus identification in the late 1800s. The initial school of thought maintained that electrical stimulation served primarily to produce, rather than prevent, epileptiform activity. One of the earliest reports of direct cortical electrical stimulation came from Rushton Parker and Francis Gotch in 1893.[1] To localize and resect a presumed motor cortex seizure focus responsible for refractory, debilitating complex partial seizures in a 9-year-old boy, characterized by hand and arm "fits," the authors performed intraoperative stimulation of the motor cortex via a single burrhole. As reported by Parker in the *British Medical Journal*, "Stimulation of the cortex at one point evoked movements of the thumb, and at an adjacent point movements of the wrist. The areas thus stimulated were scooped out with a sharp spoon..."[1]

For the better part of the early 20th century, electrical stimulation was used for seizure induction in animal models of epilepsy. In 1957, Chapman and colleagues[2] reported results of human electrical stimulation via depth electrodes placed in the amygdala of six patients with presumed temporal lobe epilepsy. Patients were stimulated 4 to 6 days after implantation, with 10, 20, or 60 pulses per second, 1-ms pulse duration, at 6 to 20 V. The authors made two useful observations: (1) depth electrode spikes were not always accompanied by scalp electroencephalogram (EEG) spikes, and (2) certain levels of stimulation seemed to induce auras similar to those experienced before seizures but not actual seizures. The first observation set the stage for understanding both the limitations of scalp EEG and the potential held by implanted depth electrodes in gathering a unique set of localized electrographic data. The second observation suggested electrical stimulation is capable of modifying endogenous activity.

Animal studies in the 1960s provided further evidence that brief pulses of direct cortical stimulation were capable of modulating underlying neuronal activity, without causing an epileptiform response.[3,4] The hypothesis that low-level stimulation could actually modulate abnormal neuronal activity was tested in small case series of deep brain stimulation (DBS) in patients with refractory epilepsy. Few studies were published in the early 1980s showing a modest effect on seizure reduction with DBS of the cerebellum and anterior thalamus.[5–7] For the next 20 years, data for DBS in various, mostly limbic anatomic locations thought responsible for epilepsy continued to come in the form of small case series, until the SANTE trial (Stimulation of the Anterior Nucleus of

Dr Robert Goodman serves as a consultant for NeuroPace, Inc.
[a] Department of Neurological Surgery, Columbia University, 710 West 168th street, New York, NY 10032, USA
[b] Department of Neurological Surgery, St Luke's-Roosevelt, 1000 Tenth Avenue, Suite 5 G-80, New York, NY 10019, USA
* Corresponding author.
E-mail address: pg2223@columbia.edu

Thalamus for Epilepsy) was initiated in 2005. The SANTE trial was the first large-scale, randomized, controlled trial for DBS of the anterior thalamus in patients with medically refractory partial epilepsy. Recently published results showed a mean seizure frequency percent reduction of 40.4% in the stimulated group versus 14.5% in the control group (compared with a preimplant baseline) at the end of the 3-month blinded phase. Long-term follow-up, including all stimulated patients beyond the blinded phase, showed a mean seizure frequency reduction of 41% at 13 months and 56% at 25 months.[8] This particular type of DBS for seizure reduction is considered a form of open loop stimulation, wherein electrical current is applied independent of endogenous electrical activity. The physicians set the stimulation parameters via an external programmer. When turned on, the electrical current continues at defined settings irrespective of any clinical or electrographic seizure activity.

Responsive Neurostimulation

With the advent of computing technology, the idea emerged that exogenous electrical stimulation could be programmed to occur in response to endogenous electrographic events, termed *closed loop stimulation*. In 1991, Nakagawa and Durand[9] described one of the earliest models of experimental responsive neurostimulation in a model of spontaneous epileptiform activity from rat hippocampi bathed in high concentrations of potassium. The authors designed a two-step algorithm that detected the onset of epileptiform activity from the hippocampus through defining a voltage derivative threshold, and immediately delivered a programmable current via stimulation electrodes. The authors were able to suppress 100% of interictal bursts in 90% of hippocampal slices. Intracellular recordings suggested that the mechanism of suppression was through hyperpolarization of the somatic membrane via the applied current, resulting in suppression of neuronal firing. Several years later, Lesser and colleagues[10] provided evidence suggesting that pulsed stimulation in humans could significantly decrease afterdischarges. The authors reported that patients receiving cortical stimulation using subdural electrodes for pre-resection evaluations often developed afterdischarges, and that brief bursts of pulse stimulation could abort and significantly decrease the duration of these discharges. These data were the first to support the hypothesis that electrical stimulation could be used to abort seizures in humans.

The first completely implantable closed-loop device developed for investigational use in humans is called the RNS System (NeuroPace,

Inc, Mountain View, California). The device was designed to record electrocorticographic (ECoG) activity and use seizure-detection algorithms to deliver responsive stimulation via implanted electrodes. The device consists of a combination of one or two subdural and/or depth electrodes surgically implanted at the epileptogenic zones, connected to the neurostimulator. The neurostimulator is a programmable, battery-powered microprocessor that is placed in a full-thickness craniectomy. Physicians are able to set detection and stimulation parameters using a programmer with a telemetry interface. The programmer also allows physicians to retrieve ECoG data from the device, a remote monitor allows the patient to retrieve data from the device, and a computerized patient data management system stores retrieved data. Because the implanted neurostimulator has a limited capacity to store data, the computerized management system allows physicians to download and save long-term data.

The RNS System, like other surgical epilepsy interventions, was intended for use in patients with medically refractory epilepsy. Other surgical interventions predating responsive neurostimulation in development include anterior temporal lobectomy, selective focus resection, amygdalo-hippocampectomy, vagus nerve stimulation, and DBS. Compared with resective procedures, stimulation devices have the advantages of reversibility and modifiability, with the goal of causing no permanent injury to functional tissue. The RNS has an additional benefit over open-loop devices such as the vagus nerve stimulator and DBS, because it is capable of recording chronic ECoG data that may be useful for seizure focus localization, counts, and characterization. In particular, the RNS may be useful in patients with bitemporal epilepsy to determine laterality,[11,12] and long-term ambulatory recordings with invasive electrodes have the potential to provide data that may be useful in resective planning. Furthermore, the device has the potential to provide patients with warning of an electrical seizure onset before the actual clinical onset occurs.

The RNS device has been under investigation since early results from patients enrolled in a phase I feasibility study were first reported at the 2004 American Epilepsy Society meeting. Vossler and colleagues[13] reported their findings from four patients supporting the safety and potential efficacy of the device. Initial data regarding the device's efficacy were later provided in an interim report of 24 patients. The investigators described a responder rate (>50% decrease in seizure frequency) of 43% for complex partial seizures and 35% for total disabling seizures.[14]

The RNS pivotal trial was then initiated and subsequently presented at the 2009 American Epilepsy Society meeting. The trial was designed to be similar to other surgical epilepsy trials (in particular, the SANTE trial) as a randomized double-blind clinical trial, enrolling 191 patients with medically refractory epilepsy at 32 centers. Patients were randomized to stimulation or no stimulation for 12 weeks, beginning 8 weeks after device implantation. Of the 191 patients with medically refractory partial-onset epilepsy who underwent implantation, those in the treatment group (responsive stimulation active) experienced a mean reduction of 37.9% in their disabling seizures compared with 17.3% for those in the placebo stimulation group (responsive stimulation inactive) ($P<.012$) during the blinded evaluation period.[15]

At the 2010 American Epilepsy Society meeting the long-term follow-up results from the RNS feasibility study and the pivotal trial were presented. A total of 256 subjects were implanted, with a mean age of 34 years, mean number of anti-epileptic drugs of 2.9, and a median seizure frequency of 10.1 seizures per 28 days. The median percent reduction in seizure frequency after 2 years postimplant was greater than 40% and the responder rate was greater than 45%. A responder rate of 53% was seen after 3 years, suggesting that the reduction in seizure frequency provided by the device has a sustained effect in this patient population.[16] No difference was seen in adverse events between the treatment and sham groups, including an overall incidence of infection (2.6%) and extradural hematoma (1%). No changes in mood or neuropsychiatric testing occurred. Final results of the comprehensive RNS pivotal trial are accepted for publication and an application for FDA approval is being pursued.

Neurostimulation in epilepsy has witnessed a century-long evolution that began with cortical stimulation in an attempt to reproduce seizure activity, and progressed to the determination through experimental models that neurostimulation could be used to both modulate and suppress abnormal neuronal firing. The recent development of advanced responsive stimulation via a closed-loop device (the RNS System) has provided evidence that epilepsy treatment continues to move toward the possibility of reducing or eliminating seizures in medically refractory patients.

REFERENCES

1. Parker R. A case of focal epilepsy: trephining: electrical stimulation and excision of focus: primary healing: improvement. Br Med J 1893;1:1101–3.

2. Chapman WP, Singh MM, Schroeder HR, et al. Temporal lobe epilepsy: brief review; responses on electrical stimulation of the amygdaloid region in six patients. Am J Med 1957;23:107–19.

3. Bindman LJ, Lippold OC, Redfearn JW. The action of brief polarizing currents on the cerebral cortex of the rat (1) during current flow and (2) in the production of long-lasting after-effects. J Physiol 1964;172:369–82.

4. Denney D, Brookhart JM. The effects of applied polarization on evoked electro-cortical waves in the cat. Electroencephalogr Clin Neurophysiol 1962;14:885–97.

5. Wright GD, McLellan DL, Brice JG. A double-blind trial of chronic cerebellar stimulation in twelve patients with severe epilepsy. J Neurol Neurosurg Psychiatry 1984;47:769–74.

6. Upton AR, Amin I, Garnett S, et al. Evoked metabolic responses in the limbic-striate system produced by stimulation of anterior thalamic nucleus in man. Pacing Clin Electrophysiol 1987;10:217–25.

7. Cooper IS, Upton AR, Amin I. Reversibility of chronic neurologic deficits. Some effects of electrical stimulation of the thalamus and internal capsule in man. Appl Neurophysiol 1980;43:244–58.

8. Fisher R, Salanova V, Witt T, et al. Electrical stimulation of the anterior nucleus of thalamus for treatment of refractory epilepsy. Epilepsia 2010;51:899–908.

9. Nakagawa M, Durand D. Suppression of spontaneous epileptiform activity with applied currents. Brain Res 1991;567:241–7.

10. Lesser RP, Kim SH, Beyderman L, et al. Brief bursts of pulse stimulation terminate afterdischarges caused by cortical stimulation. Neurology 1999;53:2073–81.

11. Gigante P, Goodman R. Chronic ambulatory EEG findings via implanted device prior to unilateral resection for bitemporal seizures. Presented at the American Society for Stereotactic and Functional Neurosurgery Biennial Meeting. New York, June 13–16, 2010.

12. Spencer D, Gwinn R, Salinsky M, et al. Laterality and temporal distribution of seizures in patients with bitemporal independent seizures during a trial of responsive neurostimulation. Epilepsy Res 2011;93:221–5.

13. Vossler D, Doherty M, Goodman R, et al. Early safety experience with a fully implanted intracranial responsive neurostimulator for epilepsy. Presented at the 58th Annual Meeting of the American Epilepsy Society Meeting. New Orleans, December 3–7, 2004.

14. Sun FT, Morrell MJ, Wharen RE Jr. Responsive cortical stimulation for the treatment of epilepsy. Neurotherapeutics 2008;5:68–74.

15. Morrell MJ, RNS System Pivotal Investigators. Results of a multicenter double blinded randomized

controlled pivotal investigation of the RNS(TM) system for treatment of intractable partial epilepsy in adults. Presented at the 63rd Annual American Epilepsy Society Meeting. Boston, December 4–8, 2009.

16. Heck CN. Long term follow-up of the RNS (TM) system in adults with medically intractable partial onset seizures. Presented at the 64th Annual American Epilepsy Society Meeting. San Antonio, December 3–7, 2010.

Responsive Neurostimulation Suppresses Synchronized Cortical Rhythms in Patients with Epilepsy

Vikaas S. Sohal, MD, PhD[a,b,c],*, Felice T. Sun, PhD[d]

KEYWORDS
- Synchrony • Gamma rhythms • Phase locking • Stimulation
- Neocortex • Hippocampus

Well established as a modality for the treatment of Parkinson disease, deep brain stimulation and other direct stimulations of neural tissues are increasingly being investigated to treat several neurologic and psychiatric conditions, including epilepsy (for review see[1]), depression,[2] obsessive-compulsive disorder,[3,4] and Tourette syndrome.[5] Despite this increasing potential clinical utility, the mechanisms by which deep brain stimulation and other forms of neurostimulation, including electroconvulsive therapy, transcranial magnetic stimulation, and vagus nerve stimulation, modulate neuronal activity remain unknown. Deep brain stimulation and other forms of intracranial neurostimulation require mechanistic explanation at multiple levels: (1) how does neurostimulation affect directly stimulated neurons and their processes, (2) how do these direct local effects of stimulation acutely affect patterns of large-scale activity in populations of neurons, and (3) how do these effects ultimately alter macroscopic

activity in brain regions over the long term. Recent work suggests that deep brain stimulation in the subthalamic nucleus may alleviate the symptoms of Parkinson disease by exciting axons from distant, possibly cortical, structures.[6] Imaging work suggests that in depression, deep brain stimulation in axons near the subgenual cingulate (Cg25) may ultimately lead to downregulation of activity in the Cg25 and consequent changes in other interconnected regions.[7] In this article, we focus on how intracranial neurostimulation affects synchronous rhythmic activity in populations of neurons. Disrupting synchronous activity may be an important therapeutic mechanism for deep brain stimulation in Parkinson disease[8] and is also likely to be critically important for the treatment of epilepsy, which is, almost by definition, characterized by abnormal neural synchrony. We describe the effects of neurostimulation on rhythmic activity recorded intracranially from the neocortex and hippocampus in patients

---

Disclosure: V.S. Sohal was a paid consultant for NeuroPace, Inc from 2006 until 2010. F.T. Sun is an employee of NeuroPace, Inc.

V.S. Sohal is supported by the Staglin Family and the International Mental Health Research Organization (IMHRO).

[a] Department of Psychiatry, University of California, San Francisco, 401 Parnassus Avenue, San Francisco, CA 94127, USA
[b] Keck Center for Integrative Neuroscience, University of California, San Francisco, 401 Parnassus Avenue, San Francisco, CA 94127, USA
[c] Sloan-Swartz Center for Theoretical Neurobiology, University of California, San Francisco, San Francisco, CA 94127, USA
[d] NeuroPace, Inc, 1375 Shorebird Way, Mountain View, CA 94043, USA
* Corresponding author.
E-mail address: vikaas.sohal@ucsf.edu

with epilepsy participating in a clinical investigation of an implantable responsive neurostimulation (RNS) system (RNS System, NeuroPace, Inc, Mountain View, CA, USA). We found that responsive stimulation acutely suppresses phase locking between gamma-frequency rhythmic activities recorded at different locations.

METHODS
Electrocorticographic Recordings

Electrocorticographic (ECOG) signals were recorded from 65 patients participating in a feasibility clinical trial of the responsive stimulation System. This was a multicenter trial conducted between 2004 and 2007 designed to demonstrate adequate safety and provide preliminary evidence for effectiveness. The trial was approved by the Food and Drug Administration and investigational review boards of each center, and informed consent was obtained from all patients.

The responsive stimulation System provides responsive cortical stimulation via a cranially implanted programmable neurostimulator connected to 1 or 2 recording and stimulating depth and/or subdural cortical strip leads that are surgically placed in the brain according to the seizure focus. The neurostimulator continually senses ECOG activity and is programmed by the physician to detect abnormal ECOG activity and then provide stimulation. Forty-one subjects had leads implanted in the neocortex, 19 had leads implanted in the hippocampus, and 5 had leads implanted in the hippocampus and neocortex. In total, 95 patients had leads located in the neocortex, and 29 had leads in the hippocampus. Two channels of bipolar recordings were available for each lead. Whenever recording sites or the recording montage changed, data from that patient were treated as a new data set, resulting in 146 data sets.

The cranially implanted neurostimulator processes the signals in real time, using detection parameters that were unique to each patient and adjusted over time to detect epileptiform activity. When stimulation was enabled, detection events were followed after a short latency (typically 60–300 microseconds) by electrical stimulation (typically high frequency; >90% of stimulation occurred at frequencies between 100 and 333 Hz, delivered pulses that were 120–200 microseconds wide, and lasted 100–200 milliseconds). ECOG records (sampled at 250 Hz and typically 60–180 seconds in duration) were stored in response to preprogrammed events (such as an individual detection event or multiple consecutive detection events).

Selection of ECOG Data

Some ECOG records contained multiple detection events, each of which would be followed by stimulation if stimulation was enabled. To minimize effects from one stimulation that might affect the analysis of later stimuli, we only analyzed data corresponding to the first stimulation event in each ECOG record. The wavelet analyses described later occurred at discrete time points, which were defined relative to the detection event. In ECOG records containing responsive stimulation, these time points were always measured relative to the detection event immediately preceding the stimulation. This measurement allowed us to compare activity at corresponding time points in ECOG records that contained stimulation (after detection events) and those containing detection events only. During the period immediately following stimulation, signals could be saturated or blanked (ie, no signal available for analysis) or contain transient low-frequency (<1 Hz) artifacts. To ensure that our results were not affected by these sorts of stimulation artifacts, we verified that ECOG signals from every recording channel were nonzero and nonsaturated throughout a window surrounding each time point. This window was large enough to include all time points that might contribute to the analysis via temporal filtering and the wavelet transformation. Any ECOG records that did not meet these criteria were excluded from the analysis. We only analyzed data sets in which a minimum of 10 ECOG records with and without stimulations were available to calculate the phase-locking statistic.

Wavelet Analysis

To study rhythmic activity, we first computed the discrete wavelet transform of activity in each channel at each time point. We based our analysis on a previously described approach.[9] Specifically, for each frequency, f, we first band-pass filtered recordings between $f \pm 2.5$ Hz (**Fig. 1**B) and then convolved the filtered signal with a wavelet of frequency f to obtain an amplitude and a phase given by

$$e^{-t^2/2\sigma^2} e^{2\pi if} \tag{1}$$

where $\sigma = 4/3f$ and f is the frequency.

Measuring Phase Locking

Following the approach described by Lachaux and colleagues,[9] we used phases obtained from the discrete wavelet transformation described earlier to calculate a measure of phase locking. For each pair of recordings from each data set, we computed phase differences, converted these to unit vectors in the complex plane (see **Fig. 1**C),

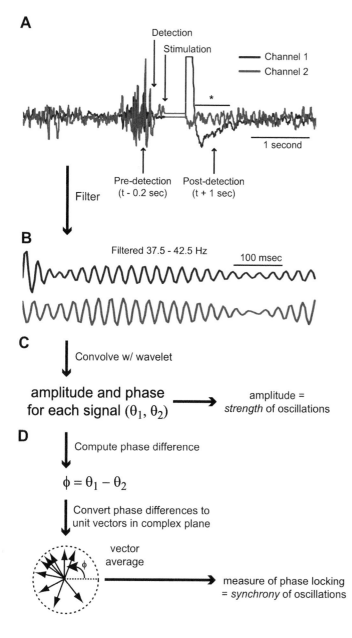

A

Detection

Stimulation

—— Channel 1
—— Channel 2

*

1 second

Pre-detection   Post-detection
(t - 0.2 sec)   (t + 1 sec)

Filter

B

Filtered 37.5 - 42.5 Hz

100 msec

C

Convolve w/ wavelet

amplitude and phase
for each signal (θ_1, θ_2)

amplitude =
strength of oscillations

D

Compute phase difference

$\phi = \theta_1 - \theta_2$

Convert phase differences to
unit vectors in complex plane

ϕ

vector
average

measure of phase locking
= *synchrony* of oscillations

Fig. 1. Overview of responsive stimulation and data analysis. (*A*) ECOG signals were recorded using chronically implanted intracranial electrodes. Signals were processed in real time to detect epileptiform activity. When epileptiform activity was detected and the stimulation was enabled, detections were followed by high-frequency electrical stimulation, as shown (of note, the sensing amplifiers were blanked during the brief period of stimulation). To determine acute effects of stimulation, we compared signals 1.0, 0.5, and 0.2 seconds before and 1.0, 1.2, and 2.0 seconds after detection events with stimulation with signals before and after detection events in the absence of stimulation. (*B*) To analyze activity at a particular frequency, we band-pass filtered each signal around that frequency, before convolving with a wavelet to obtain the amplitude and phase at that frequency. (*C, D*) To compute phase locking between a pair of signals, for each ECOG record, we computed the phase difference for those 2 signals and converted all the phase differences (corresponding to different ECOG records) to unit vectors in the complex plane. The amplitude of the vector average of all these vectors measured phase locking.

and used the amplitude of the average of these unit vectors to measure the degree of phase locking or synchrony at frequency *f*. We refer to this measure as the phase-locking statistic.

Determination of Statistically Significant Phase Locking

We determined whether a particular value of the phase-locking statistic was statistically significant using bootstrapping. Specifically, we computed 1000 random values of the phase-locking statistic. Each of these was the sum of N unit vectors in the complex plane, each of which had a pseudorandom phase. N is the number of phases (or unit vectors) that was used to calculate the original phase-locking statistic. Then, we obtained a *P* value by determining how often the actual calculated phase-locking statistic exceeded these pseudorandom values of the phase-locking statistic.

RESULTS

We studied how responsive stimulation affected rhythmic activity in the neocortex and hippocampus. As described in the "Methods" section, ECOG signals were recorded from chronically implanted intracranial electrodes in patients with epilepsy. Briefly, a cranially implanted neurostimulator continually senses ECOG activity and detects abnormal ECOG activity. If stimulation was enabled, detection events were followed after a short latency by electrical stimulation. Brief ECOG records were stored containing detection events (with and without stimulation). **Fig. 1A** shows ECOG data from 2 distinct channels recorded simultaneously during a detection event followed by stimulation.

To study rhythmic activity, we measured both the amplitude of rhythmic activity and the degree of phase locking, or synchrony, between rhythmic activities recorded simultaneously from different channels, based on a previously described approach.[9] The detailed method for computing this measure of phase locking, referred to as the phase-locking statistic, is described in the "Methods" section. This measure of phase locking is similar to coherence, but does not require stationary signals, and measures the phase relationship independent of amplitude. We compared the strength and synchrony of oscillations 1.0, 0.5, and 0.2 seconds before detection events and 1.0, 1.2, and 2.0 seconds after these events. As described in the "Methods" section, we omitted data containing stimulation artifacts. We measured the statistical significance of phase locking by bootstrapping as described in the "Methods" section. We analyzed frequencies between 10 and 100 Hz in 5-Hz intervals, although in some cases we then grouped frequencies into 4 bands: 10 to 30 Hz representing alpha and beta bands, 35 to 50 Hz representing low-gamma band, 55 to 80 Hz representing the mid-gamma band, and 85 to 100 Hz representing the high-gamma band. Low frequencies (<10 Hz) were excluded because of the potential amplifier-sensing artifact, whereas high frequencies (>100 Hz) were excluded because recordings included a low-pass analog filter of approximately 80 to 90 Hz to minimize aliasing for signals lower than 125 Hz.

To study the effects of responsive stimulation on phase locking, we focused on those ECOG records containing statistically significant phase locking ($P<.05$) either before or after detection events (with and without stimulation). The presence of phase locking was similar in ECOG records containing stimulations (16.8% of all electrode pairs exhibited phase locking) and those containing detection events that were not followed by stimulations (16.3% of all electrode pairs exhibited phase locking). This fraction was much higher than would be expected by chance (9%). To compare changes in phase locking that occur after rhythmic stimulation with those occurring after detection events in the absence of stimulation, we looked at data

collected from the same patients, using the electrode configurations, in which both the ⟨ lation and detection-only data sets con⟨ statistically significant phase locking at the frequency. There were 239 such cases, and⟨ were drawn from 60 data sets (out of 12⟨ data sets).

Fig. 2 shows phase locking, as a function ⟨ relative to the detection event, for these ⟨ (stimulation present vs detection events Note that the phase-locking statistic ca⟨ between 0 (no phase locking) and 1 (perfect locking). Both the data containing stimulatior data containing detection events only show a⟨ rise in phase locking from 500 to 200 millise⟨ preceding the detection event and an event⟨ turn to the baseline level of phase locking. Ho⟨ after stimulations, the phase-locking 1 secon⟨ the detection event decreases by an aver⟨ $-8\% \pm 4\%$. By contrast, in the absence of st⟨ tion, the phase locking continues to rise, ⟨ average of $3\% \pm 4\%$. As a result, the phase l⟨

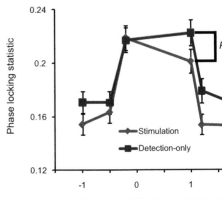

Fig. 2. Responsive stimulation acutely suppresse⟨ locking. The phase-locking statistic is plotted as ⟨ tion of time, averaged over all cases (ie, a pa⟨ frequency and electrode pair from a particula⟨ set), which showed statistically significant phase ⟨ in both ECOG records containing stimulations an⟨ containing detections only. We calculated the ⟨ locking statistic at 6 time points: 1.0 second, 0.5 s⟨ and 0.2 seconds before the detection event a⟨ second, 1.2 seconds, and 2.0 seconds after the de⟨ event. In the events with responsive stimulation ⟨ lations were delivered shortly after the detectio⟨ (ie, within 300 milliseconds). There is a sharp ris⟨ phase-locking statistic between 0.5 and 0.2 s⟨ before the detection event. After stimulatio⟨ phase-locking statistic drops, whereas in ECOG ⟨ containing detections only, the phase-locking ⟨ continues to rise, such that the phase-locking ⟨ is significantly different in these 2 cases ($P<.05$, ⟨ t test). Error bars = ± 1 standard error of the me⟨

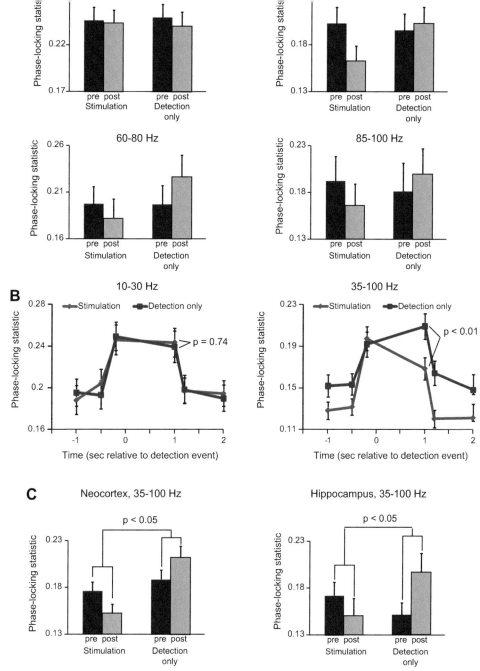

Fig. 3. The effects of responsive stimulation are frequency dependent. (*A*) Comparison of the phase-locking statistic 0.2 seconds before and 1.0 second after detection events (pre and post, respectively) for various frequency bands and for ECOG records that contain stimulation events or contain detection events only. There is a significant interaction between the frequency band (10–30 vs 35–100 Hz) and the condition (stimulation vs detection-only) on the change in phase locking (post-pre) ($P<.05$ by analysis of variance), that is, stimulation suppresses the phase-locking statistic for gamma-frequency (35–100 Hz) activity but not lower-frequency (10–30 Hz) activity. (*B*) The phase-locking statistic over time for activity in the alpha and beta frequency bands (10–30 Hz, *left*) and the gamma-frequency band (35–100 Hz, *right*). As in **Fig. 2**, data are averaged over all cases (ie, a particular frequency and electrode pair from a particular data set), which showed statistically significant phase locking in both ECOG records containing stimulations and those containing detections only. (*C*) Comparison of the phase-locking statistic 0.2 seconds before and 1.0 second after detection events for gamma-frequency activity recorded from the neocortex (*left*) or hippocampus (*right*). In both regions, stimulation suppresses gamma-frequency phase locking. Error bars = ±1 standard error of the mean.

is significantly lower after stimulations than in the absence of stimulation ($P<.05$; 2-tailed t test).

We then looked at the change in phase locking after stimulation versus detection only as a function of frequency (**Fig. 3**A). The effects of stimulation on phase locking seem to occur throughout the gamma-frequency range (35–100 Hz) but not at lower frequencies (10–30 Hz). There was a statistically significant interaction between frequency band (10–30 vs 35–100 Hz) and the presence of stimulation on the change in phase locking (see **Fig. 3**B; $P<.05$ by 2-way analysis of variance): stimulation reduces gamma-frequency (35–100 Hz) phase locking measured 1 second after the detection event by 15% $\pm$ 7%, whereas in the absence of stimulation, gamma-frequency phase locking actually increases by 20% $\pm$ 5% ($P<.01$ for a difference in the change in phase locking after stimulation vs after detection only; 2-tailed t test). By contrast, the change in lower-frequency (10–30 Hz) phase locking was similar whether or not stimulation was present (change in phase locking after stimulation: -1% $\pm$ 7%, change in phase locking after detection event only: -4% $\pm$ 6%; $P = .74$ by 2-tailed t test). Moreover, the markedly different changes in gamma-frequency phase locking after stimulation versus after detection only were also found when we analyzed data from neocortical and hippocampal leads separately (see **Fig. 3**C; $P<.05$ for a difference in the change in phase locking after stimulation vs after detection only, for both hippocampal and neocortical data sets; 2-tailed t test).

We also studied how stimulation affects rhythmic amplitudes measured using our wavelet analysis (see **Fig. 1**). The mean baseline amplitude

(1 second before detection events) was different in ECOG records containing stimula and those containing detections only (74 $\pm$ 120 $\pm$ 4 arbitrary units, respectively). Ther we restricted our analysis to cases in whic a particular patient, frequency, and electrod mean amplitudes for ECOG records cont stimulations and those containing detection e only differed by less than 25% (N = 2464 cases). As with phase locking, we observed a increase in rhythmic amplitudes betweer and 200 milliseconds before detection e (**Fig. 4**A). One second after the detection amplitudes had decreased sharply regardl whether or not stimulation had occurred **Fig. 4**A). We observed a similar pattern ever restricting analysis to rhythmic activity i gamma-frequency range from electrodes exhibit statistically significant phase locking **Fig. 4**B). We also observed a similar pattern we normalized amplitudes, relative to all a tudes recorded from the same channel. although detection events seem to be prec and followed by sharp changes in the ampl of rhythmic activity, we did not find evidenc responsive stimulation affects these change

DISCUSSION

We found that responsive stimulation a (ie, within 1 second) suppresses the long synchrony of gamma-frequency rhythmic act intracranial ECOG data. Long range ref synchronization between distinct leads, as op to local synchrony of activity recorded at a location. Notably, this long-range sync

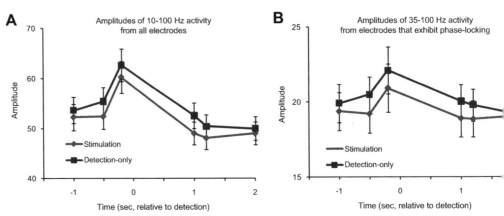

Fig. 4. Responsive stimulation does not produce clear effects on rhythmic amplitudes. (*A*) Rhythmic amp obtained via the wavelet transformation, over time, averaged over all cases (ie, a particular frequency ar trode from a particular data set), which contained at least 10 ECOG records in each condition (stimulation vs detection only). (*B*) Rhythmic amplitudes over time, now restricted to cases that exhibited statistically cant phase locking and frequencies in the gamma range (35–100 Hz).

measured using the phase-locking statistic, rises sharply during the second preceding detection events and continues to rise in the absence of stimulation. The phase-locking statistic remains depressed 2 seconds after the detection event, suggesting that the effects of responsive stimulation are not transient. Rather, responsive stimulation seems to accelerate the return of the phase-locking statistic to baseline after the detection of epileptiform activity.

We initially focused on phase locking, quantified in a way that is independent of the amplitude of 2 signals, because there is the possibility that amplifier gain could be compromised immediately after stimulation because of effects such as saturation. However, the wavelet analysis we used did measure rhythmic amplitudes, and, although we observed sharp changes in rhythmic amplitudes before and after the detection of epileptiform activity, we did not find consistent effects of stimulation on these amplitude changes.

Relationship with Possible Therapeutic Mechanisms of Deep Brain Stimulation

Although we did not directly measure the clinical consequences of these effects, a decrease in long-range rhythmic synchrony almost by definition corresponds to a decrease in epileptiform activity. These effects represent clinical evidence for the hypothesis that deep brain stimulation reduces pathologic cortical synchrony[10] and may be related to the observation that responsive stimulation is most effective during particular phases of an afterdischarge.[11] These effects may also explain how deep brain stimulation could potentially disconnect the site of stimulation from downstream targets[7] because synchronized oscillations may mediate communication between brain regions. Changes in phase locking were confined to the gamma-frequency band, which is thought to be particularly important for communication between cortical regions.[12–14]

LIMITATIONS

As described in the "Methods" and "Results" sections, we have tried to control for possible confounders in several ways. First, we focused on phases, rather than amplitudes, which could be affected by amplifier saturation. Second, we studied the effects of stimulation 1 second after a detection event in order to minimize electronic artifacts related to stimulation. Third, we bandpass filtered our signals to eliminate low-frequency artifacts of stimulation. In particular, the observed changes in phase locking at high, but not low, frequencies suggest that our results do not reflect such artifacts. Fourth, we compare changes in phase locking after stimulation with those that occur after detection events in the absence of stimulation in order to focus on true effects of stimulation rather than regression to the mean and other factors related to the intrinsic evolution of neural signals after a detection event.

Despite these efforts, several possible confounders remain. ECOG records containing detection events, but not stimulations, are not perfect controls for ECOG records containing stimulations because in many cases these were recorded from the same patients with the same electrode and lead configurations but at different times. Furthermore, even though we only analyzed effects of the first stimulation in each ECOG record, ECOG records containing stimulations are likely to have occurred in the context of other stimulations. As a result, the acute effects of stimulation that we describe should be interpreted in the context of possible subacute and chronic effects of stimulation. We studied the effects of stimulation on phase locking by restricting our analysis to the subset of cases (activity at a particular frequency, that occurred in a particular electrode pair, from a particular patient) that exhibited statistically significant phase locking. As described earlier, these cases represent a small fraction of the total data collected. Of course, our data are limited in that we could only sample from the locations where electrodes were implanted and leads were placed. Thus, it is possible that stimulation had an effect on many phase-locked oscillations in the brain that we could not detect. In addition, as mentioned earlier, in order to avoid impact from stimulation artifacts, we did not analyze signals for 1 second after the detection event. It is possible that by doing so, we missed some acute effects of stimulation or underestimated the magnitude of the stimulation-induced suppression of phase locking, which seems to decay over time (see **Fig. 2**). An inherent limitation is that electrodes were implanted in epileptogenic regions. Thus, our results are limited to analysis of such regions and may not necessarily reflect effects of neurostimulation in or on other regions.

SUMMARY

We found that responsive stimulation acutely (eg, within 1 second) suppresses phase-locked oscillations in the neocortex and hippocampus of patients with epilepsy. These results suggest a specific mechanism by which responsive stimulation could suppress epileptiform activity and disconnect stimulated regions from downstream targets, possibly contributing to the therapeutic effects of neurostimulation in epilepsy and other neuropsychiatric conditions.

ACKNOWLEDGMENTS

We thank the editors of *Neurosurgery Clinics* and the guest editors of this special issue for inviting this submission.

REFERENCES

1. Saillet S, Langlois M, Feddersen B, et al. Manipulating the epileptic brain using stimulation: a review of experimental and clinical studies. Epileptic Disord 2009;11(2):100–12.
2. Mayberg HS, Lozano AM, Voon V, et al. Deep brain stimulation for treatment-resistant depression. Neuron 2005;45(5):651–60.
3. Greenberg BD, Malone DA, Friehs GM, et al. Three-year outcomes in deep brain stimulation for highly resistant obsessive-compulsive disorder. Neuropsychopharmacology 2006;31(11):2384–93.
4. Nuttin B, Gybels J, Cosyns P, et al. Deep brain stimulation for psychiatric disorders. Neurosurg Clin N Am 2003;14(2):xv–xvi.
5. Visser-Vandewalle V, Temel Y, Boon P, et al. Chronic bilateral thalamic stimulation: a new therapeutic approach in intractable Tourette syndrome. Report of three cases. J Neurosurg 2003;99(6):1094–100.
6. Gradinaru V, Mogri M, Thompson KR, et al. Optical deconstruction of parkinsonian neural circuitry. Science 2009;324(5925):354–9.
7. Johansen-Berg H, Gutman DA, Behrens TE, et al. Anatomical connectivity of the subgenual cingulate region targeted with deep brain stimulation for treatment-resistant depression. Cereb Cortex 2008; 18(6):1374–83.
8. Hauptmann C, Tass PA. Therapeutic rewiring by means of desynchronizing brain stimulation. Biosystems 2007;89(1–3):173–81.
9. Lachaux JP, Rodriguez E, Martinerie J, et al. Measuring phase synchrony in brain signals. Hum Brain Mapp 1999;8(4):194–208.
10. Popovych OV, Hauptmann C, Tass PA. Effective desynchronization by nonlinear delayed feedback. Phys Rev Lett 2005;94(16):164102.
11. Motamedi GK, Lesser RP, Miglioretti DL, et al. Optimizing parameters for terminating cortical afterdischarges with pulse stimulation. Epilepsia 2002; 43(8):836–46.
12. Rodriguez E, George N, Lachaux JP, et al. Perception's shadow: long-distance synchronization of human brain activity. Nature 1999;397(6718): 430–3.
13. Womelsdorf T, Schoffelen JM, Oostenveld R, et al. Modulation of neuronal interactions through neuronal synchronization. Science 2007;316(5831): 1609–12.
14. Sohal VS, Zhang F, Yizhar O, et al. Parvalbumin neurons and gamma rhythms enhance cortical circuit performance. Nature 2009;459(7247):698–702.

Seizure Prediction and its Applications

Leon D. Iasemidis, PhD[a,b,c],*

KEYWORDS

- Spatiotemporal dynamical analysis of EEG • Ictogenesis
- Seizure prediction • Closed-loop seizure control

Epilepsy is considered a window to the brain's function and is therefore an increasingly active, interdisciplinary field of research.[1,2] The sacred or divine disease is among the most common disorders of the nervous system, second only to stroke and Alzheimer disease, and affects 1% to 2% of the world's population.[3,4] Although epilepsy occurs in all age groups, the highest incidences occur in infants and in the elderly.[5–7] This high incidence of epilepsy stems from it having a large number of causes, including genetic abnormalities, developmental anomalies, and febrile convulsions, as well as brain insults such as craniofacial trauma, central nervous system infections, hypoxia, ischemia, and tumors.

The hallmarks of epilepsy are recurrent seizures and epileptic spikes. If seizures cannot be controlled, the patient experiences major limitations in family, social, educational, and vocational activities. These limitations have profound effects on the patient's quality of life.[8] Epileptic seizures and spikes are caused by the sudden development of pathologic, synchronous neuronal firing in the cerebrum and can be recorded by scalp, subdural, and intracranial electrodes. Seizures may begin locally in portions of the cerebral hemispheres (partial/focal seizures) with a single or multiple foci, or simultaneously in both cerebral hemispheres (generalized seizures). After a seizure's onset, partial seizures may remain localized and cause mild cognitive, psychic, sensory, motor, or autonomic symptoms, or may spread (secondarily generalized) to cause altered consciousness, complex automatic behaviors, or bilateral tonic-clonic convulsions. Even though seizures typically run their course (seconds to minutes) and the brain subsequently recovers by itself, there are cases in which recovery is accomplished only through external intervention (ie, high doses of antiepileptic drugs), as in status epilepticus (SE), a life-threatening condition.[9,10] The brain also does not recover by itself in the event of sudden unexplained death in epilepsy (SUDEP). SUDEP is a less common condition than SE, is seemingly unpredictable, and hence extremely difficult to monitor and provide for external intervention.[11,12]

One of the most debilitating aspects of epilepsy is that seizures seem to occur without warning. Until recently, the general belief in the medical community was that epileptic seizures could not be anticipated. Seizures were assumed to occur abruptly and randomly over time. However, hypotheses on the mechanisms of ictogenesis and predictability of seizures had been postulated in the past based on reports from clinical practice (eg, existence of auras) and scientific intuition (eg, theory of reservoir).[13,14] In the 1970s, attempts to show that seizures are predictable had also been undertaken via computer analysis of the electroencephalogram (EEG).[15] Despite those early attempts, the results were not encouraging. Systematic and robust detection of a preictal period across seizures in the same patient, as

---

The author has nothing to disclose.

[a] The Harrington Department of Biomedical Engineering, School of Biological and Health Systems Engineering, Arizona State University, PO Box 879709, Tempe, AZ 85287-9709, USA

[b] Department of Electrical Engineering, School of Electrical, Computer and Energy Engineering, Arizona State University, PO Box 875706, Tempe, AZ 85287-5706, USA

[c] Department of Neurology, Mayo Clinic, 5777 East Mayo Boulevard, Phoenix, AZ 85054, USA

* Corresponding author. The Harrington Department of Biomedical Engineering, School of Biological and Health Systems Engineering, Arizona State University, PO Box 879709, Tempe, AZ 85287-9709.

E-mail address: iasemidis@asu.edu

Neurosurg Clin N Am 22 (2011) 489–506

doi:10.1016/j.nec.2011.07.004

well as across patients, remained elusive. The essential features of the brain's transition to epileptic seizures were not captured, and a theoretic framework for seizure development that could lead to definition and subsequent detection of such preictal features was missing.[16,17]

It was in the 1980s that new signal processing methodologies emerged, based on the mathematical theory of nonlinear dynamics and chaos for the study of spontaneous formation of organized spatial, temporal, or spatiotemporal patterns in physical, chemical, and biologic systems.[18–29] These methodologies quantified the complexity and randomness of the signal from the perspective of invariants of nonlinear dynamics and represented a drastic departure from the signal processing techniques based on linear systems analysis (eg, Fourier analysis). Because the brain is inherently a nonlinear system, the general concept at that time was that seizures represented transitions of the epileptic brain from its normal, less ordered (chaotic) state to an abnormal, more ordered state and back to a normal state along the lines of chaos-to-order-to-chaos transitions.[30] How this concept, when applied to the EEG in epilepsy, eventually changed some long-held beliefs about seizures and their dynamical causes is discussed later. Within this framework, systematic mathematical analysis of long-term EEG recordings that included seizures started in the mid-1980s at the University of Michigan (U of M), creating, at the time, the largest worldwide database of digitally stored peri-ictal EEG recordings with seizures. The existence of long-term preictal periods (order of minutes) was shown in 1988 by nonlinear dynamical analysis of EEGs recorded by subdural arrays from patients undergoing phase II monitoring of their seizures at the U of M Hospital's Epilepsy Monitoring Unit (EMU).[31]

EXISTENCE OF A PREICTAL PERIOD: SEIZURE PREDICTABILITY

Among the important measures of the dynamics a linear or nonlinear system exhibits are the Lyapunov exponents that measure the average information flow (bits per second) the system produces along local eigendirections in its state space.[32,33] Positive Lyapunov exponents denote generation of information, whereas negative exponents denote destruction of information. A chaotic nonlinear system possesses at least 1 positive Lyapunov exponent, and it is because of this feature that its behavior seems random, even if it is deterministic in nature. Methods for calculating these measures of dynamics from experimental data have been published.[34]

The brain, being nonstationary, is never in a steady state in the strictly dynamical sense, at any location. We have shown that, in the case of a nonstationary system with transients like epileptic spikes, the use of the short-term maximum Lyapunov exponent (STL_{max}) constitutes a more accurate characterization of the rate of the average information flow[35] than the traditional maximum Lyapunov (L_{max}) exponent.[36] STL_{max} is estimated from sequential EEG segments of 10 seconds in duration per recording site to create a set of STL_{max} profiles with time. Analysis of scalp, subdural, or depth EEG from patients with focal (temporal and frontal lobe) epilepsy at the U of M, and subsequently at the University of Florida and Arizona State University, showed that the STL_{max} profiles at brain sites systematically and progressively converge to similar values tens of minutes before a seizure and remain entrained up to the onset of the seizure.[37–48] We have called this phenomenon preictal dynamical entrainment (convergence of measures of EEG dynamics long before a seizure onset), the involved brain sites critical sites, and the corresponding pairs of sites that interact in this dynamical sense critical pairs. The focal sites are typically part of the set of critical sites. Therefore, the following hypothesis was formed that directly relates to mechanisms of ictogenesis: the epileptic brain is dynamically entrained by the focal sites long before a seizure's occurrence.

It was further hypothesized that the brain starts malfunctioning because of this loss of relative independence of processing of information at normal brain sites long before a seizure develops. Such a preictal entrainment is illustrated in **Fig. 1** for a patient with focal epilepsy and EEG recorded by intracranial electrodes (see **Fig. 1**A, B). The STL_{max} profiles of critical sites with time are shown in **Fig. 1**C. The convergence of STL_{max} profiles of a pair of sites is quantified by the T-index, a statistical measure of the distance between the mean values of the respective time series. Small values of T-index denote small distances between the corresponding STL_{max} profiles, and hence entrainment of dynamics. T-index values with time are estimated within a running window of 10 minutes in duration (60 STL_{max} values) for a pair of STL_{max} profiles. Pairs of sites that are dynamically entrained in the 10-minute period before a seizure are characterized as critical pairs. The average T-index profile illustrated in **Fig. 1**D represents the average of all T-indices over time across the thus selected critical pairs of sites. From **Fig. 1**D, it is clear that, if critical pairs of sites are selected (retrospectively) from the immediate preictal period of a seizure, a seizure is predictable. For example, in the seizure depicted in **Fig. 1**B, a warning

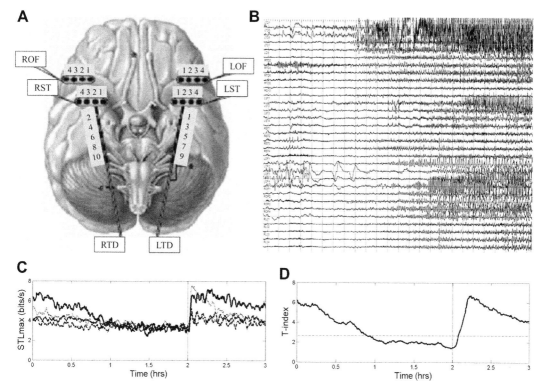

Fig. 1. Detection of long preictal periods and resetting of brain dynamics at seizures. (*A*) The electrode montage used for recording of intracranial EEG. LOF, left orbitofrontal; LST, left subtemporal; LTD, left hippocampus; ROF, right orbitofrontal; RST, right subtemporal; RTD, right hippocampus. (*B*) A typical electrographic onset of seizures for a patient with focal temporal lobe epilepsy (25 seconds of EEG is shown around a seizure's onset, band-pass analog filtered between 0.5 and 70 Hz, and then sampled at 200 Hz and stored digitally on hard drive). The seizure was secondarily generalized and lasted for 2.5 minutes. The epileptogenic focus was determined as RTD. (*C*) STL_{max} profiles from 2 hours before to 1 hour after seizure's onset at RST4 (solid line), LOF2 (dotted line), RTD8 (dashed line), and LTD9 (dotted/dashed line) electrodes. (*D*) The average T-index profile was estimated by averaging the T-indices of the critical electrode pairs (in this seizure, 119 out of a total of 435 possible electrode pairs). The critical pairs selected are the ones that are dynamically entrained 10 minutes before the electrographic seizure's onset (retrospective calculation; ie, test of seizure predictability). Values of T-index below the horizontal dotted line at 2.662 in the T-index plot denote dynamical entrainment (statistical convergence of the corresponding pairs of the STL_{max} profiles at the $\alpha = 0.01$ significance level). The vertical dotted lines in panels (*C*) and (*D*) denote the seizure's onset (at about 2 hours into the recording). It is clear that (1) preictal entrainment of critical brain sites was reversed to disentrainment following seizure onset, and (2) if those critical electrode pairs had been prospectively followed since the beginning of the recording, a warning for the impending seizure could have been issued at the onset of the preictal period, that is, about 1 hour before this seizure's occurrence.

could have been issued about 1 hour before its onset (see **Fig.** 1D), that is, when the average T-index crosses the statistical threshold $T_{th} = 2.662$ ($\alpha = 0.01$ significance level for convergence of STL_{max} profiles) from above.[47]

Other measures of dynamics, like phase, also exhibit dynamical entrainment in the preictal period, although later than STL_{max}.[49–51] In addition to patients, epileptic rats with chronic epilepsy also exhibit measurable preictal periods in the order of minutes.[52–58] These results show that seizures are not abrupt transitions in and out of an abnormal ictal state, but instead they follow a dynamical transition that may evolve for minutes to hours. During this preictal dynamical transition, multiple regions of the brain progressively approach a similar dynamical state. Because such spatiotemporal transitions are progressive with time, it has been suggested that, in addition to preictal periods, seizure susceptibility periods could also be identified from analysis of corresponding interictal profiles of brain dynamics.[59]

RESETTING OF BRAIN DYNAMICS AT SEIZURES

Seizures typically reset the preictal dynamical entrainment and lead to the disentrainment of dynamics of the focus from the rest of the brain. This important conjecture can be observed by comparing the average T-index values and their trend in the preictal period versus the postictal period. For example, after seizure's onset (see **Fig. 1**D), there is a trend toward disentrainment of the preictally entrained pairs of sites (T-index moves rapidly toward higher values above T_{th} and toward ones it exhibited before the beginning of the preictal period). **Fig. 1**C shows the same trend at the level of STL_{max} profiles of individual brain sites. We have called this reversal of dynamics brain resetting at seizures and we have observed it in focal as well as generalized seizures, within and across patients.[60–66] We also have observed it using other measures of brain dynamics.[67] Furthermore, the observed dynamical resetting in patients with epilepsy is significantly specific to seizures at the $\alpha = 0.05$ statistical significance level.[64] Other groups have independently observed similarly reversal trends using classic methods of signal processing.[68,69] This observation may reflect a passive mechanism (eg, high electrical activity during a seizure depletes critical neurotransmitters and thus deactivates critical neuroreceptors in the entrained neuronal network). An alternative explanation is an active mechanism, that is, seizure activity releases neuropeptides that may subsequently contribute to the temporary repair of a pathologic feedback network (discussed later) that allowed the dynamical entrainment to occur and to last for tens of minutes. Such an explanation is analogous to mechanisms attributed to seizures associated with electroconvulsive therapy (ECT).[70,71]

Given the resetting of the brain's pathological entrainment with the focus at seizures, and the recovery that follows, one would expect that seizures in SE fail to reset this pathology of brain dynamics. Indeed, we have observed this after a similar to the above dynamical analysis of the EEG from patients with SE in the emergency room (ER), intensive care unit (ICU), or the EMU.[72,73] Successful antiepileptic drug (AED) administration, which interrupted SE seizures in rats and humans, resulted in the resetting of brain dynamics. Unsuccessful AED administration in humans and/or no AED administration in SE rats failed to reset the brain dynamics, with lethal consequences. Thus, resetting of dynamics could be used to monitor treatment of SE by AEDs, as well as for the evaluation of current AEDs, and possibly the design of new AEDs. Psychogenic nonepileptic seizures do not seem to reset the brain dynamics, and the phenomenon of resetting could thus be used as a tool for differential diagnosis between epileptic and psychogenic nonepileptic seizures.[74]

SEIZURE PREDICTION

The ability to identify a mathematically defined preictal period via dynamical analysis of EEG and seizure predictability studies has constituted the basis for implementation of algorithms for prospective prediction of epileptic seizures.[75–83] A major difficulty encountered in the attempt to prospectively predict an impending seizure is illustrated in **Fig. 2**. In this figure, the average T-index profiles created from critical pairs of dynamically entrained sites in the 10 minute interval prior to 3 different time instants (1.45 hours, 0.57 hours, and 0 hours before seizure onset) are shown for a second typical seizure from the same patient as in **Fig. 1**. It is evident that, if critical pairs are selected far away from that seizure (see **Fig. 2**A), they may not be the relevant ones for prediction of this seizure. For example, critical pairs selected from 1.45 hours before seizure onset become disentrained before the seizure's occurrence, whereas pairs selected from within the preictal period of this seizure are kept entrained until the seizure occurs to disentrain them. (The preictal period is defined and estimated from the average T-index profile of critical pairs selected in the 10 minute interval prior to 0 hours before seizure onset; see **Fig. 2**C.) The participation of the epileptogenic focus in the critical sites in each case is illustrated in **Fig. 3**. Visual inspection of **Fig. 3**A, B shows that participation of the focus (right hippocampus in this patient) in the entrainment of normal sites becomes prominent as the seizure approaches. Thus, monitoring the T-index profile of the relevant critical pairs of sites is of paramount importance for prospective seizure prediction. The solution we have given to this problem is adaptive optimal estimation of critical sites (first-generation seizure prediction algorithms[80]) or pairs of sites (second-generation seizure prediction algorithms, independent from user input and without need for optimization from training datasets, that is, ready to run anytime on any patient without any a priori information[81]). In each case, predetermined rules are applied for adaptive selection of the critical sites or pairs of sites over time from present and past T-index values. These seizure prediction algorithms, applied to scalp and/or intracranial EEG from patients and/or animals with epilepsy, have achieved greater than 80% sensitivity (that is, more than 80% of seizures are predicted), fair specificity (false prediction rate of 0.12–0.17 per hour, that is, 1 false positive per 8 to 7 hours respectively) and average prediction time of more than 45 minutes per seizure (that is, issue of a warning for an impending seizure 45 minutes before its occurrence). Sensitivity and specificity did not depend on either seizure rate or the recording EEG modality.

Following our first findings on seizure predictability, there have been many investigations by

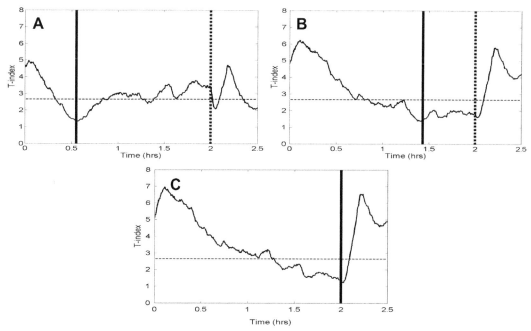

Fig. 2. Selection of relevant critical brain sites/pairs is important for seizure prediction. Supportive analysis is here shown around a second seizure from the same patient as in **Fig. 1**B. (*A*) Average T-index profile from critical pairs (all pairs that were identified to be statistically entrained with respect to their STL$_{max}$ measures of dynamics) within a 10-minute interval about 1.45 hours (left vertical line in this panel) before the onset (right dotted vertical line) of a seizure. The number of critical pairs thus identified was 120 and did not all remain entrained up to the seizure. (*B*) Average T-index profile from critical pairs of brain sites within a 10-minute interval about 0.57 hours (left vertical line in this panel) before the onset (right vertical dotted line) of the seizure. The number of critical pairs thus identified was 161, remained entrained up to the seizure, and were disentrained postictally. (*C*) Average T-index profile from critical pairs of brain sites within a 10-minute interval immediately before the seizure's onset (therefore, left and right vertical lines in this panel coincide). The number of critical pairs thus identified was 168 and, with retrospective evaluation, they became entrained about 40 minutes before this seizure's onset (therefore, preictal period = 40 minutes here). From this figure, it is clear that (1) there are different critical pairs entrained at different times before a seizure, (2) a progressive entrainment of critical sites can be observed as a seizure approaches only if relevant critical sites are selected, and (3) for a seizure prediction scheme to be successful, adaptive estimation of critical brain sites relevant to the upcoming seizure has to be performed over time.

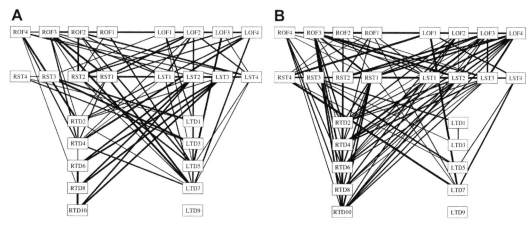

Fig. 3. Topography of preictal dynamical entrainment: Network connectivity maps from analysis of brain dynamics at instances long before a seizure. In these maps, 2 brain sites are shown connected if they are dynamically entrained for 10 minutes before the instance at which the map is generated. Because our measures of dynamics (STL$_{max}$) are estimated every 10 seconds, connectivity maps can be produced every 10 seconds. (*A*) Brain connectivity map generated 1.45 hours before the seizure in **Fig. 2**, which is still in the interictal period (see **Fig. 2**A). (*B*) Brain connectivity map generated 0.57 hours before the seizure; that is, in the preictal period of this seizure (see **Fig. 2**B and **Fig. 2**C). The seizure focus is in the right hippocampus (right vertical column in the graphs) and it seems that, as seizure approaches (transition from interictal to preictal period), the pathologic right takes over the more normal left hippocampus in the dynamical entrainment of the rest of the brain.

other research groups worldwide in the last 20 years. References, chronologically cited herein from 1990 to 2010, indicate these investigations.[84–183] A variety of methods have been used in analysis of short-term and long-term EEG: parametric (model based) or nonparametric (transform based), linear or nonlinear, reference dependent (eg, using baseline EEG segments from interictal periods) or independent, and at the microscopic (neuronal) or macroscopic (network) level. In general, these investigations have pointed to seizure predictability with varying degrees of success. Methods for statistical evaluation of their performance, regarding sensitivity and specificity on training and testing EEG datasets, also against periodic or pseudorandom warning time series, and the use of surrogate data to account for spurious values and noise in the EEG have been developed.[184–205] However, on seizure prediction (prospective analysis) few investigations have been performed. Seizure prediction, which is what is needed in medical applications, is different from and more difficult to achieve than seizure predictability, as we have argued and shown earlier. A more recent investigation in seizure prediction was performed by Schulze-Bonhage's group, a group that was very skeptical in the past with respect to feasibility of seizure prediction schemes.[206] These investigators reported a maximum mean sensitivity of 43.2%, at a false seizure prediction rate of 0.15 per hour. Training on each patient's EEG data was required before a prospective run of the algorithm on a patient. The interval at which a seizure was predicted ahead of time was not clearly reported but appeared to be in the range of 10 to 60 minutes. Although this performance is sensitivity-wise almost half of what we have reported in the past, even with our first-generation seizure prediction algorithms,[80] it is an additional piece of independent evidence that seizures can not only be predictable (retrospective analysis) but predicted (prospective analysis) too.

Most recently, two other groups have attempted prospective seizure prediction using pattern recognition methodologies.[207,208] A training stage per patient was required here too. The reported specificity values varied widely per patient while sensitivity to seizures was very high and appeared encouraging. However, in a closer inspection, both groups used the Freiburg database,[201] that is, a database with fragmented, discontinuous EEG data (one 24 hour interictal period well separated from about 50 min preictal periods for a couple of seizures per patient). Even though this is an intermediate step towards seizure prediction, it may give a false picture of the capabilities of a seizure prediction algorithm, which has to work not only in real time but on line on continuous EEG data. This fact is shown by Freiburg group's recent publication[206] and the poor results they obtained about sensitivity using a fair specificity value when they decided to run their algorithms on long-term continuous EEG data.

APPLICATION OF SEIZURE PREDICTION TO SEIZURE CONTROL

Incorporation of seizure prediction algorithms to neuromodulation schemes for abatement of seizures is one important area of application in the modern treatment of epilepsy (eg, via electromagnetic stimulation as in DBS, VNS, TDC and TMS, and via implantable cooling or in situ chemicals release/drug delivery systems).[209–211] Our findings from analysis of long-term EEG dynamics in the domains of seizure predictability, prediction, and resetting, in animals and patients with various types of epileptic seizures and EEG recordings (scalp and intracranial), led us to formulate the following hypothesis about ictogenesis in terms of basic principles of control in adaptive linear or nonlinear dynamical systems: epileptic seizures may occur because of pathologic alterations in the global and/or local internal feedback loops in the brain, normally responsible for keeping the spatial correlations (interactions, synchronizations/entrainment) within strict limits with respect to time and space in order to support the brain's fast multiprocessing and multitask function.

Using neuronal population models that are capable of exhibiting seizurelike behavior, we have shown that entrainment (disentrainment) of the populations' STL_{max}, with increased (decreased) coupling between populations, resembles the observed preictal dynamical entrainment (postictal disentrainment) of the STL_{max} at critical sites in the epileptic brain.[212,213] In agreement with burst phenomena in adaptive systems, seizures in these models occur if the existing (internal to the models) feedback loops are pathologic, in the sense that they lack the ability to compensate fast enough for excessive increases in the network coupling. This situation eventually leads to seizurelike transitions in those models. Motivated by these findings, we postulated the existence of an internal pathologic feedback action in the epileptic brain; subsequently, using a control-oriented approach, we developed a functional model for an external seizure controller. During periods of abnormally high synchrony (entrainment), the developed control scheme provides appropriate desynchronizing feedback to maintain normal synchronization levels between neural

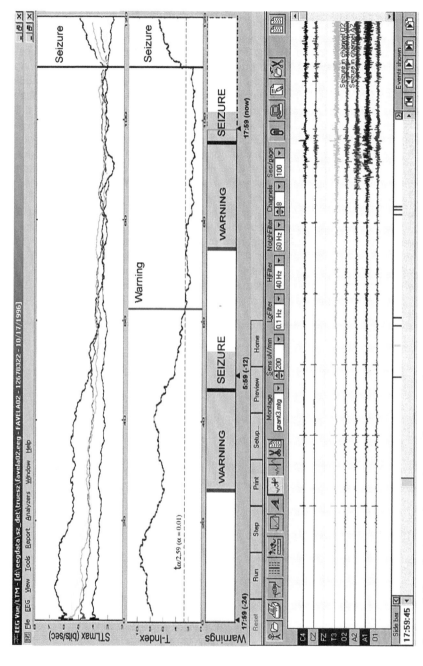

Fig. 4. Real-time online prediction of seizures. A snapshot on the screen of a personal computer that runs our second generation adaptive seizure prediction program in real time on simultaneously recorded EEG from a rat with chronic epilepsy. The 2 waveforms displayed at the top are respectively the STL_{max} and average T-index profiles generated from automatically determined critical sites over time. The profile that includes the seizure warnings and seizure occurrences is displayed in the next row (scale in HOURS). The online, real-time, recorded EEG is displayed in the last row (scale in SECONDS). (*Data from* Sabesan S. Spatiotemporal brain dynamics in epilepsy: application to seizure prediction and focus localization. PhD dissertation. Tempe (AZ): Arizona State University; 2008.)

populations (homeostasis of dynamics). We have called this closed-loop feedback control view of epileptic seizures, and the developed seizure control strategies, feedback decoupling and have validated it on coupled chaotic oscillator models and biologically plausible neurophysiologic models.[214–228]

Within the context of closed-loop, real-time, on-line control of seizures, seizures should be anticipated with good sensitivity and specificity from dynamical analysis of EEG, and effective external intervention is applied to change the pathologic brain dynamics (long-term entrainment) in a timely manner and prevent a seizure from occurring. To this end, we used our adaptive seizure prediction algorithm in the feedback branch of a closed-loop electrical stimulation scheme for seizure control. The lithium-pilocarpine (LP) model of acute SE in rats was chosen as the animal model for chronic epilepsy. Male Sprague-Dawley rats were used for the study. Three to 4 weeks after induced SE, rats were implanted with a 6 micro-wire monopolar electrodes targeted to 4 cortical and 2 hippocampal locations; 2 Teflon-coated tungsten bipolar twisted stimulating electrodes were implanted in the centromedial thalamic

nucleus. Our second-generation seizure p tion program was used to predict, online a real time, the developed seizures (**Fig. 4** trigger an A-M Systems Model 2300 stim unit (Carlsborg, WA, USA) at seizure warnin a seizure warning, a train of square pulse delivered in a charge-balanced bipolar ca fashion (**Fig. 5**).

Results from this experiment are sho **Fig. 6**. The experiment consisted of week just-in-time (closed-loop) stimulation (phas D in **Fig. 6**) and periodic (open-loop) stimu (phase E in **Fig. 6**). Weeks of dramatic red of seizures (see panel 3 in **Fig. 6**) followe in-time adaptive stimulation of the epilept focus (left hippocampus; localized by analy the EEG by focus localization algorithms until resetting of dynamics is achieved (ph in **Fig. 6**), whereas less reduction of seizure lowed just-in-time stimulation of the tha (phases A and B in **Fig. 6**). No reduction of se compared with baseline followed open-loop odic (period equal to the inverse of the m seizure rate in baseline) stimulation of the (phase E in **Fig. 6**). These results impl closed-loop, focal stimulation scheme

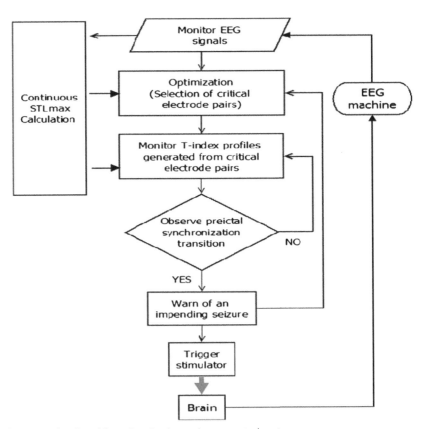

Fig. 5. Flow diagram of a closed-loop just-in-time seizure control system.

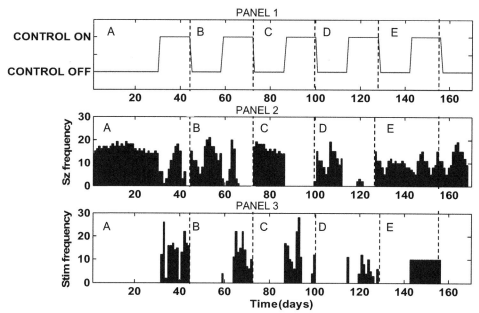

Fig. 6. Real-time control of seizures in an epileptic rat via closed-loop and open-loop deep brain stimulation (DBS). In the closed-loop seizure control scheme (just-in-time), electrical stimulus was administered at seizure warnings that were issued by our online second-generation seizure prediction program according to the flow diagram described in **Fig. 5**. In the open-loop seizure control scheme (periodic), electrical stimuli were delivered periodically without using any feedback/knowledge of the state of the concurrent brain dynamics. Both control schemes used the following traditional predefined electrical stimulus: train of periodic biphasic pulses of 130-Hz frequency, and each pulse of 200-microsecond duration (pulse-width) and 200-μA amplitude. The experiment consisted of the following 5 different phases of stimulation, each including recording of about 3 weeks of EEG with stimulation off and 3 weeks with stimulation on. The 5 different phases are schematically depicted in panel 1 of this figure: (*A*) Just-in-time, closed-loop stimulation of the thalamus for 1 minute immediately after issue of a seizure warning. (*B*) Just-in-time closed-loop stimulation of the thalamus after a seizure warning for as long as it takes (up to an upper limit) to reset the entrained critical pairs. (*C*) Just-in-time closed-loop stimulation of the focus (left hippo-campus) for 1 minute after each seizure warning. (*D*) Just-in-time closed-loop stimulation of the focus (left hippo-campus) after a seizure warning for as long as it takes (up to an upper limit) to reset the entrained critical pairs. (*E*) Periodic open-loop focal (hippocampal) stimulation for 1 minute at a time, with frequency equal to seizure frequency of the preceding to phase E baseline. The seizure frequency (# seizures per day) with time is shown in panel 2 (middle panel). The frequency of stimulation (# sets of stimulations per day) is shown in panel 3 (bottom panel) and, as expected, was variable with time for phases A–D, and constant for phase E. The most successful stim-ulation schemes in reducing seizure frequency were schemes C and D, in which seizure frequency was even reduced to zero for days at a time. The worst seizure control scheme was the periodic scheme E. Stim, stimulus; Sz, seizure. (*Data from* Sabesan S. Spatiotemporal brain dynamics in epilepsy: application to seizure prediction and focus local-ization. PhD dissertation. Tempe (AZ): Arizona State University; 2008.)

superior to closed-loop, nonfocal schemes, which in turn are superior to open-loop, focal schemes. The demonstration of the importance of incorporating seizure prediction algorithms in closed-loop control schemes (just-in-time), as well as of the location of stimulation, for online seizure abatement was one goal of this experiment. The importance of stimulus form for seizure abatement, such that it ensures resetting of the entrainment of dynamics, was another goal (use of long stimuli until dynamics are reset resulted in further reduction of seizure rates; compare phases A vs B, and C vs D in **Fig. 6**). These results are in broad agreement and better than the ones we reported in Ref.[228] with the epileptogenic focus identifica-tion and adaptive stimulation of the focus (hippo-campus) versus thalamus contributing a lot to the observed drastic improvement in seizure abatement.

A LOOK INTO THE FUTURE

The results from investigations into seizure predic-tion in the last 25 years have established firm foun-dations for direct clinical applications to epilepsy.[231] The concepts delineated in this article constitute the basis for a dynamical interpretation of ictogenesis and lead to long-term prediction of seizures tens of minutes before their clinical or electrographic onset, detection of seizure susceptibility periods, and the development of innovative treatments for epilepsy through timely interventions to control seizure occurrence (eg, via electrical stimulation and/or in situ drug delivery). We have shown that timing of intervention is critical for successful control of seizures, and that seizure prediction algorithms can now provide this important information online and in real time, making them an important component of future brain pacemakers for epilepsy.

Seizures seem to be the end result of a progressive recruitment of brain sites by the focus toward an abnormal synchronization of dynamics. The onset of such recruitment occurs on the order of minutes with respect to seizure prediction, on the order of hours and days with respect to seizure susceptibility. Resetting of this pathologic preictal dynamical recruitment occurs at seizures. In cases in which seizures are unable to reset this disorder of dynamics (eg, in SE), external intervention (eg, via AEDs) may be successful.

In light of the previous discussion, a dynamical systems perspective of the epileptic brain can also be formulated. Seizures could result from the inability of internal feedback mechanisms to provide timely compensation/regulation of coupling (entrainment) between brain sites, and hence seizure control may be achieved by preictally and/or interictal decoupling the pathologic sites via externally provided appropriate feedback. Such optimal feedback decoupling has been found to be a function of both the recorded EEGs and the coupling between respective brain sites.[220,221,226,227] According to this hypothetical dynamical scheme of ictogenesis, the following series of events has been conjectured: (1) brain in spatiotemporal chaos; (2) internal or external stimulus enters the system and changes the spatial coupling between two or more brain sites; (3) spatial coupling produces spatial correlations, possibly storing the information about the stimulus and/or initiating action; (4) spatial correlations activate an internal compensating feedback mechanism; (5) compensation tries to remove (or assimilate) the developed spatial correlations; (6) the system returns to spatiotemporal chaos if step 5 is successful. In the normal brain, the correlations in the network must lie within a normal range and vary quickly in response to a stimulus, which implies that the internal feedback path should be well tuned and able to track changes of the coupling with time reasonably well. In the epileptic brain, step 5 involves pathologic (poorly

tuned) internal feedback paths. The observed long-term dynamical entrainment before seizures can then be interpreted as an indicator of disorder in the internal feedback of the network. According to the theory of adaptive systems control, such disorders can exhibit large errors in the estimation of the coupling, and in turn cause local destabilization and bursting of the network (seizures). This rationale can also be applied to explain the mechanisms of reflex epilepsies, with external stimuli as inputs to the system causing enduring entrainment, and seizures following to reset it.

A global view of epilepsy and seizures in terms of systems dynamics and control theory constitutes an interdisciplinary avenue of research between engineering, neuroscience, and medicine, and has already shown that it can generate refreshing results and novel hypotheses. I strongly believe that it would benefit the epilepsy patient if this path continues to be pursued and developed further in the years to come.

ACKNOWLEDGMENTS

I would like to acknowledge the support of this research by the National Institutes of Health (NIH EB002089 BRP Grant on Brain Dynamics; NIH SBIR 1R43NS050931-01A1; NIH R21 NS061310-01A1), the Epilepsy Research Foundation of America and Ali Paris Fund for LKS Research, the National Science Foundation (grant no. 0,601,740), and the Arizona Science Foundation (Competitive Advantage Award grant CAA 0281-08).

REFERENCES

1. Temkin O. The falling sickness: a history of epilepsy from the Greeks to the beginnings of modern neurology. 2nd edition. Baltimore (MD): Johns Hopkins University Press; 1994.
2. Lockard JS, Ward AA, editors. Epilepsy: a window to brain mechanisms. New York: Raven Press; 1992.
3. Engel J Jr, Pedley TA, editors. Epilepsy: a comprehensive textbook. Philadelphia: Lippincott Williams & Wilkins; 1998.
4. Cascino GD, Sirven JI, editors. Adult epilepsy. Hoboken (NJ): John Wiley & Sons; 2011.
5. Hauser WA, Kurland LT. The epidemiology of epilepsy in Rochester, Minnesota, 1935 through 1967. Epilepsia 1975;16:1–66.
6. Forsgren L. Prospective incidence study and clinical characterization of seizures in newly referred adults. Epilepsia 1990;31:292–301.
7. Begley CE, Heaney DC. The economic burden of epilepsy. Epilepsia 2002;43:S4.

8. Goldstein MA, Harden CL. Continuing exploration of the neuropsychiatry of seizures: a review of anxiety and epilepsy. Epilepsy Behav 2000;1:228–34.

9. Fountain NB. Status epilepticus: risk factors and complications. Epilepsia 2000;41:23–30.

10. Claassen J, Lokin JK, Fitzsimmons BF, et al. Predictors of functional disability and mortality after status epilepticus. Neurology 2002;58:139–42.

11. Tomson T, Nashef L, Ryvlin P. Sudden unexpected death in epilepsy: current knowledge and future directions. Lancet Neurol 2008;7(11):1021–31.

12. Sperling MR. Sudden unexplained death in epilepsy. Epilepsy Curr 2001;1:21–3.

13. Penfield W. The evidence for a cerebral vascular mechanism in epilepsy. Ann Int Med 1993;7:303–10.

14. Lennox WG. Science and seizures. New York: Harper; 1946.

15. Viglione S, Walsh G. Proceedings: epileptic seizure prediction. Electroencephalogr Clin Neurophysiol 1975;39(4):435–6.

16. Rogowski Z, Gath I, Bental E. On the prediction of epileptic seizures. Biol Cybern 1981;42:9–15.

17. Lange HH, Lieb JP, Engel J Jr, et al. Temporospatial patterns of preictal spike activity in human temporal lobe epilepsy. Electroencephalogr Clin Neurophysiol 1983;56:543–55.

18. Babloyantz A, Destexhe A. Low dimensional chaos in an instance of epilepsy. Proc Natl Acad Sci U S A 1986;83:3513–7.

19. Glass L, Goldberger AL, Courtemanche M, et al. Nonlinear dynamics, chaos and complex cardiac arrhythmias. Proc R Soc Lond 1987;413:9–26.

20. Rensing L, An der Heiden U, Mackey MC. Temporal disorders in human oscillatory systems. Berlin: Springer-Verlag; 1987.

21. Degn H, Holden A, Olsen LF. Chaos in biological systems. New York: Plenum; 1987.

22. Bai-Lin H. Chaos. Singapore: World Scientific; 1987.

23. Freeman WJ. Simulation of chaotic EEG patterns with a dynamic model of the olfactory system. Biol Cybern 1987;56:39–150.

24. Skarda CA, Freeman WJ. How brains make chaos in order to make sense of the world? Behav Brain Sci 1987;10:161–95.

25. Mayer-Kress G, Layne SP. Dimensionality of the human electroencephalogram. Ann N Y Acad Sci 1987;504:62–87.

26. Kelso JAS, Mandel AJ, Shlesinger MF. Dynamical patterns in complex systems. Singapore: World Scientific; 1988.

27. Marcus M, Aller SM, Nicolis G. From chemical to biological organization. Berlin: Springer-Verlag; 1988.

28. Milton JG, Longtin A, Beuter A, et al. Complex dynamics and bifurcations in neurology. J Theor Biol 1989;138:29–147.

29. Baker G, Gollub J. Chaotic dynamics. Cambridge (MA): Cambridge University Press; 1990.

30. Iasemidis LD. Epileptic seizure prediction and control. IEEE Trans Biomed Eng 2003;50(5):549–58.

31. Iasemidis LD, Zaveri HP, Sackellares JC, et al. Nonlinear dynamics of electrocorticographic data. J Clin Neurophysiol 1988;5:339.

32. Sackellares JC, Iasemidis LD, Zaveri HP, et al. Inference on the chaotic behavior of the epileptogenic focus. Epilepsia 1989;29:682.

33. Iasemidis LD, Sackellares JC, Zaveri HP, et al. Phase space topography of the electrocorticogram and the Lyapunov exponent in partial seizures. Brain Topogr 1990;2:187–201.

34. Iasemidis LD, Sackellares JC. The temporal evolution of the largest Lyapunov exponent on the human epileptic cortex. In: Duke DW, Pritchard WS, editors. Measuring chaos in the human brain. Singapore: World Scientific; 1991. p. 49–82.

35. Iasemidis LD. On the dynamics of the human brain in temporal lobe epilepsy [PhD dissertation]. Ann Arbor (MI): University of Michigan; 1991.

36. Wolf A, Swift JB, Swinney L, et al. Determining Lyapunov exponents from a time series. Physica D 1985;16:285–317.

37. Iasemidis LD, Sackellares JC. Long time scale spatio-temporal patterns of entrainment in preictal ECoG data in human temporal lobe epilepsy. Epilepsia 1990;31:621.

38. Iasemidis LD, Barreto A, Gilmore RL, et al. Spatiotemporal evolution of dynamical measures precedes onset of mesial temporal lobe seizures. Epilepsia 1994;35(Suppl 8):133.

39. Iasemidis LD, Pappas KE, Gilmore RL, et al. Preictal entrainment of a critical cortical mass is a necessary condition for seizure occurrence. Epilepsia 1996;37(Suppl 5):90.

40. Iasemidis LD, Sackellares JC. Chaos theory and epilepsy. Neuroscientist 1996;2:118–26.

41. Iasemidis LD, Principe JC, Sackellares JC. Spatiotemporal dynamics of human epileptic seizures. In: Harrison RG, Weiping L, Ditto W, et al, editors. Proceedings of the 3rd Experimental Chaos Conference. Singapore: World Scientific; 1996. p. 26–30.

42. Iasemidis LD, Pappas KE, Gilmore RL, et al. Detection of the preictal transition state in scalp-sphenoidal recordings. Electroencephalogr Clin Neurophysiol 1997;103(4):32P.

43. Iasemidis LD, Principe JC, Czaplewski JM, et al. Spatiotemporal transition to epileptic seizures: a nonlinear dynamical analysis of scalp and intracranial EEG recordings. In: Lopes da Silva F, Principe JC, Almeida LB, editors. Spatiotemporal models in biological and artificial systems. Amsterdam: IOS Press; 1997. p. 81–8.

44. Sackellares JC, Iasemidis LF, Shiau DS, et al. Detection of the preictal transition from scalp EEG recordings. Epilepsia 1999;40(Suppl 7):176.

45. Sackellares JC, Iasemidis LD, Gilmore R, et al. Epilepsy – when chaos fails. In: Lehnertz K, Arnhold J, Grassberger P, et al, editors. Chaos in the brain? Singapore: World Scientific; 2000. p. 112–33.

46. Iasemidis LD, Shiau DS, Pardalos P, et al. Transition to epileptic seizures – an optimization approach into its dynamics. In: Du DZ, Pardalos PM, Wang J, editors. Discrete Mathematical Problems with Medical Applications. DIMACS series. Providence (RI): American Mathematical Society Publishing Co; 2000. p. 55–74.

47. Iasemidis LD, Pardalos P, Sackellares JC, et al. Quadratic binary programming and dynamical system approach to determine the predictability of epileptic seizures. J Comb Optim 2001;5:9–26.

48. Iasemidis LD, Pardalos PM, Sackellares JC, et al. Global optimization approaches to reconstruction of dynamical systems related to epileptic seizures. In: Massalas CV, editor. Mathematical methods in scattering theory and biomedical technology. Singapore: World Scientific; 2002. p. 308–18.

49. Iasemidis LD, Shiau DS, Pardalos PM, et al. Phase entrainment and predictability of epileptic seizures. In: Pardalos PM, Principe J, editors. Biocomputing. Kluwer; 2002. p. 59–84.

50. Chaovalitwongse W, Iasemidis LD, Prasad A, et al. Seizure prediction by dynamical phase information from the EEG. Epilepsia 2002; 43:45.

51. Sabesan S, Good L, Chakravarthy N, et al. Global optimization and spatial synchronization changes prior to epileptic seizures. In: Alves CJ, Pardalos PM, Vicente LN, editors. Optimization in medicine, Springer series in optimization and its applications. Coimbra (Portugal): Springer; 2005. p. 103–25, 2008.

52. Carney PR, Iasemidis LD, Pardalos P, et al. Predictability of seizures in an epilepsy-prone transgenic mouse model. Epilepsia 2001;42(Suppl 7):225.

53. Carney PR, Maze MF, Shiau DS, et al. State specific nonlinear neurodynamical features in an animal model of generalized epilepsy. Epilepsia 2002;43:270.

54. Shiau DS, Sackellares JC, Iasemidis LD, et al. Nonlinear approximate entropy analysis of brain electrical activity in a generalized epilepsy animal model. Epilepsia 2002;43:273–4.

55. Carney PR, Shiau DS, Pardalos PM, et al. Nonlinear neurodynamical features in an animal model of generalized epilepsy. In: Pardalos PM, Sackellares JC, Carney PR, et al, editors. Quantitative neuroscience. Series on biocomputing, vol. 2. Kluwer; 2004. p. 37–51.

56. Chaovalitwongse W, Pardalos PM, Sackellares JC, et al. Applications of global optimization and dynamical systems to prediction of epileptic seizures. In: Pardalos PM, Sackellares JC, Carney PR, et al, editors. Quantitative neuroscience. Series on biocomputing, vol. 2. Kluwer; 2004. p. 1–35.

57. Sackellares JC, Iasemidis LD, Shiau DS, et al. Spatiotemporal transitions in temporal lobe epilepsy. In: Pardalos PM, Sackellares JC, Carney PR, et al, editors. Quantitative neuroscience. Series on biocomputing, vol. 2. Kluwer; 2004. p. 223–37.

58. Nair SP, Shiau DS, Iasemidis LD, et al. Seizure predictability in an experimental model of epilepsy. In: Pardalos P, Boginski V, Vazacopoulos A, editors. Data Mining in Biomedicine. Springer Series on Optimization and its Applications. New York: Springer; 2007. p. 535–58.

59. Sackellares JC, Iasemidis LD, Shiau DS, et al. Seizure susceptibility predicted by EEG dynamics. Ann Neurol 1999;52(S2):A106.

60. Sackellares JC, Iasemidis LD, Gilmore RL, et al. Epileptic seizures as neural resetting mechanisms. Epilepsia 1997;38(S3):189.

61. Shiau DS, Luo Q, Gilmore RL, et al. Epileptic seizures resetting revisited. Epilepsia 2000;41(S7):208–9.

62. Sackellares JC, Iasemidis LD, Pardalos PM, et al. Combined application of global optimization and nonlinear dynamics to detect state resetting in human epilepsy. In: Pardalos PM, Principe J, editors. Biocomputing. Boston: Kluwer Academic Publishers; 2002. p. 140–58.

63. Iasemidis LD, Prasad A, Sackellares JC, et al. On the prediction of seizures, hysteresis and resetting of the epileptic brain: insights from models of coupled chaotic oscillators. In: Bountis T, Pneumatikos S, editors. Order and chaos, vol. 8. Thessaloniki (Greece): Publishing House of K. Sfakianakis; 2003. p. 283–305.

64. Iasemidis LD, Shiau DS, Sackellares JC, et al. Dynamical resetting of the human brain at epileptic seizures: application of nonlinear dynamics and global optimization techniques. IEEE Trans Biomed Eng 2004;51:493–506.

65. Prasad A, Iasemidis LD, Sabesan S, et al. Dynamical hysteresis and spatial synchronization in coupled nonidentical chaotic oscillators. Indian Academy of Sciences. Pramana J Physics, Indian Academy of Sciences 2005;64:513–23.

66. Sabesan S, Chakravarthy N, Tsakalis K, et al. Measuring resetting of brain dynamics at epileptic seizures: application of global optimization and spatial synchronization techniques. J Comb Optim 2009;17:74–97.

67. Sabesan S, Iasemidis LD, Tsakalis K, et al. Use of dynamical measures in prediction and control of focal and generalized epilepsy. In: Osorio I, Zaveri HP, Frei MG, et al, editors. Epilepsy, the intersection of neurosciences, biology, mathematics, engineering, and physics. CRC Press; 2011. p. 307–20.

68. Medvedev AV. Temporal binding at gamma frequencies in the brain: paving the way to epilepsy? Australas Phys Eng Sci Med 2001;24(1):37–48.

69. Medvedev AV. Epileptiform spikes desynchronize and diminish fast (gamma) activity of the brain. An

"anti-binding" mechanism? Brain Res Bull 2002; 58(1):115–28.

70. Masco D, Sahibzada N, Switzer R, et al. Electroshock seizures protect against apoptotic hippocampal cell death induced by adrenalectomy. Neuroscience 1999;91:1315–9.

71. Fink M. Electroshock revisited. Am Sci 2000;88: 162–7.

72. Good LB, Sabesan S, Iasemidis LD, et al. Brain dynamical disentrainment by anti-epileptic drugs in rat and human status epilepticus. Proceedings of the 26th IEEE EMBS Annual International Conference. September 1–4, San Francisco: 2004. p. 176–9.

73. Faith A, Sabesan S, Wang N, et al. Dynamical analysis of the EEG and treatment of human status epilepticus by anti-epileptic drugs. In: Chaovalitwongse W, Pardalos PM, Xanthopoulos P, editors. Computational neuroscience. Springer series on optimization and its applications, 38. New York: Springer Science; 2010. p. 305–16.

74. Faith A, Krishnan B, Roth A, et al. Lack of resetting of brain dynamics following psychogenic non-epileptic seizures. In: Proceedings of the IASTED International symposia on imaging and signal processing in healthcare and technology. Washington, DC; May 16–18, 2011. Calgary AB Canada: Acta Press 2011.

75. Iasemidis LD, Sackellares JC, Gilmore RL, et al. Automated seizure prediction paradigm. Epilepsia 1998;39(S6):207.

76. Iasemidis LD, Shiau DS, Chaovalitwongse W, et al. Adaptive seizure prediction system. Epilepsia 2002; 43:264–5.

77. Sackellares JC, Iasemidis LD, Pardalos PM, et al. Performance characteristics of an automated seizure warning algorithm utilizing dynamical measures of the EEG signal and global optimization techniques. Epilepsia 2001;42(S7):40.

78. Sackellares JC, Shiau DS, Iasemidis LD, et al. Can knowledge of cortical site dynamics in a preceding seizure be used to improve prediction of the next seizure? Ann Neurol 2002;52(3):S65–6.

79. Sackellares JC, Iasemidis LD, Shiau DS, et al. Dynamical dependence of seizure prediction on preceding seizures. Epilepsia 2002;43:50.

80. Iasemidis LD, Shiau DS, Chaovalitwongse W, et al. Adaptive epileptic seizure prediction system. IEEE Trans Biomed Eng 2003;50(5):616–27.

81. Sabesan S. Spatiotemporal brain dynamics in epilepsy: application to seizure prediction and focus localization [PhD dissertation]. Tempe (AZ): Arizona State University; 2008.

82. Sandeep PN, Shiau DS, Principe JC, et al. An investigation of EEG dynamics in an animal model of temporal lobe epilepsy using the maximum Lyapunov exponent. J Exp Neurol 2009;216:115–21.

83. Good LB, Sabesan S, Marsh ST, et al. Nonlinear dynamics of seizure prediction in a rodent model of epilepsy. Nonlinear Dynamics Psychol Life Sci 2010;14(5):411–34.

84. Frank GW, Lookman T, Nerenberg MAH, et al. Chaotic time series analysis of epileptic seizures. Physica D 1990;46:427–38.

85. Pijn JP, Van Neerven J, Noest A, et al. Chaos or noise in EEG signals: a dependence of state and brain site. Electroencephalogr Clin Neurophysiol 1991;79:371–81.

86. Pezard L, Martinerie J, Breton F, et al. Nonlinear forecasting measurements of multichannel EEG dynamics. Electroencephalogr Clin Neurophysiol 1994;91:383–91.

87. Elger CE, Lehnertz K. Ictogenesis and chaos. In: Wolf P, editor. Epileptic seizures and syndromes. London: J. Libbey & Co; 1994. p. 547–52.

88. Lopes da Silva FH, Pijn JP, Wadman WJ. Dynamics of local neuronal networks: control parameters and state bifurcations in epileptogenesis. Prog Brain Res 1994;102:359–70.

89. Petrosian A, Homan R. The analysis of EEG texture content for seizure prediction. In: IEEE EMBS 16th Annual International Conference. November 4, Baltimore, Maryland; 1994.

90. Lehnertz K, Elger CE. Spatio-temporal dynamics of the primary epileptogenic area in temporal lobe epilepsy characterized by neuronal complexity loss. Electroencephalogr Clin Neurophysiol 1995;95:108–17.

91. Lehnertz K, Elger CE. Neuronal complexity loss of the contralateral hippocampus in temporal lobe epilepsy: a possible indicator of secondary epileptogenesis. Epilepsia 1995;36(S4):21.

92. Scott DA, Schiff SJ. Predictability of EEG interictal spikes. Biophys J 1995;69:1748–57.

93. Hively LM, Clapp NE, Daw CS, et al. Nonlinear analysis of EEG for epileptic events. ORNL/TM-12961. Oak Ridge (TN): Oak Ridge National Laboratory; 1995.

94. Qu H, Gotman J. A seizure warning system for long term epilepsy monitoring. Neurology 1995;45:2250–4.

95. Lerner DE. Monitoring changing dynamics with correlation integrals: a case study of an epileptic seizure. Physica D 1996;97:563–76.

96. Pezard L, Martinerie J, Mueller-Gerking J, et al. Entropy quantification of human brain spatio-temporal dynamics. Physica D 1996;96:344–54.

97. Schwartzkroin PA. Origins of the epileptic state. Epilepsia 1997;38:853–8.

98. Pijn JPM, Velis DN, van der Heyden MJ, et al. Nonlinear dynamics of epileptic seizures on basis of intracranial EEG recordings. Brain Topogr 1997; 9:249–70.

99. Weinand ME, Carter P, El Saadany WF, et al. Cerebral blood flow and temporal lobe epileptogenicity. J Neurosurg 1997;86:226–32.

100. Baumgrtner C, Serles W, Leutmezer F, et al. Preictal SPECT in temporal lobe epilepsy: regional cerebral blood flow is increased prior to electroencephalography-seizure onset. J Nucl Med 1998;39:978–82.

101. Lehnertz K, Elger CE. Can epileptic seizures be predicted? Evidence from nonlinear time series analyses of brain electrical activity. Phys Rev Lett 1998;80:5019–23.

102. Lehnertz K, Widman G, Elger CE. Predicting seizures of mesial temporal and neocortical origin. Epilepsia 1998;39(S6):205.

103. Elger CE, Lehnertz K. Prediction of epileptic seizures in humans from nonlinear dynamics analysis of brain electrical activity. Eur J Neurosci 1998;10:786–9.

104. Le Van Quyen M, Adam C, Baulac M, et al. Nonlinear interdependencies of EEG signals in human intracranially recorded temporal lobe seizures. Brain Res 1998;792:24–40.

105. Martinerie JM, Adam C, Le Van Quyen M, et al. Epileptic seizures can be anticipated by nonlinear analysis. Nat Med 1998;4:1173–6.

106. Schiff SJ. Forecasting brain storms. Nat Med 1998; 4(10):1117–8.

107. Osorio I, Frei MG, Wilkinson SB. Real-time automated detection and quantitative analysis of seizures and short-term prediction of clinical onset. Epilepsia 1998;39:615–27.

108. Salant Y, Gath I, Henriksen O. Prediction of epileptic seizures from two channel EEG. Med Biol Eng Comput 1998;36:549–56.

109. Le Van Quyen M, Martinerie JM, Adam C, et al. Nonlinear analyses of interictal EEG map the brain interdependencies in human focal epilepsy. Physica D 1999;127:250–67.

110. Le Van Quyen M, Martinerie JM, Baulac M, et al. Anticipating epileptic seizures in real time by a nonlinear analysis of similarity between EEG recordings. Neuroreport 1999;10:2149–55.

111. Lehnertz K, Andrzejak RG, Mormann F, et al. Linear and nonlinear EEG analysis techniques for anticipating epileptic seizures. Epilepsia 1999; 40(S2):71.

112. Arnhold J, Grassberger P, Lehnertz K, et al. A robust method for detecting interdependencies: application to intracranially recorded EEG. Physica D 1999;134:419–30.

113. Moser HR, Weber B, Wieser HG, et al. Electroencephalograms in epilepsy: analysis and seizure prediction within the framework of Lyapunov theory. Physica D 1999;130:291–305.

114. Lachaux JP, Rodriguez E, Martinerie J, et al. Measuring phase synchrony in brain signal. Hum Brain Mapp 1999;8:94–208.

115. Kopell N, Ermentrout GB, Whittington MA, et al. Gamma rhythms and beta rhythms have different synchronization properties. Proc Natl Acad Sci USA 2000;97:1867–72.

116. Mormann F, Lehnertz K, David P, et al. Mean phase-coherence as a measure for phase synchronization and its application to the EEG of epilepsy patients. Physica D 2000;144:358–69.

117. Lehnertz K, Arnhold J, Grassberger P, et al, editors. Chaos in brain? Singapore: World Scientific; 2000.

118. Elger CE, Widman G, Andrzejak R, et al. Nonlinear EEG analysis and its potential role in epileptology. Epilepsia 2000;41(S3):34–8.

119. Quiroga RQ, Arnhold J, Lehnertz K, et al. Kullback-Leibler and renormalized entropies: applications to electroencephalograms of epilepsy patients. Phys Rev E 2000;62:8380–6.

120. Hively LH, Protopopescu VA, Gailey PC. Timely detection of dynamic changes in scalp EEG signals. Chaos 2000;10:846–75.

121. Le Van Quyen M, Adam C, Martinerie JM, et al. Spatiotemporal characterizations of nonlinear changes in intracranial activities prior to human temporal lobe seizures. Eur J Neurosci 2000;12:2124–34.

122. Petrosian A, Prokhorov D, Homan R, et al. Recurrent neural network based prediction of epileptic seizures in intra- and extracranial EEG. Neurocomputing 2000;30:201–18.

123. Lehnertz K, Andrzejak R, Arnhold J, et al. Nonlinear EEG analysis in epilepsy: its possible use for interictal focus localization, seizure anticipation and prevention. J Clin Neurophysiol 2001; 18:209–22.

124. Jerger KK, Netoff TI, Francis JT, et al. Early seizure detection. J Clin Neurophysiol 2001;18:259–68.

125. Osorio I, Harrison MAF, Lai UC, et al. Observations on the application of the correlation dimension and correlation integral to the prediction of seizures. J Clin Neurophysiol 2001;18:269–74.

126. Protopopescu VA, Hively LM, Gailey PC. Epileptic event forewarning from scalp EEG. J Clin Neurophysiol 2001;18:223–45.

127. Le Van Quyen M, Martinerie JM, Navarro V, et al. Characterizing neurodynamic changes before seizures. J Clin Neurophysiol 2001;18:191–208.

128. Le Van Quyen M, Martinerie JM, Navarro V, et al. Anticipation of epileptic seizures from standard EEG recordings. Lancet 2001;357:183–8.

129. Sunderman S, Osorio I, Frei MG, et al. Stochastic modeling and prediction of experimental seizures in Sprague-Dawley rats. J Clin Neurophysiol 2001; 18:275–82.

130. Bai O, Nakamura M, Nishida S, et al. Markov process amplitude EEG model for spontaneous background activity. J Clin Neurophysiol 2001;18: 283–90.

131. Litt B, Esteller R, Echauz J, et al. Epileptic seizures may begin hours in advance of clinical onset: a report of five patients. Neuron 2001;30:51–64.

132. Varela FJ, Lachaux JP, Rodriguez E, et al. The brainweb: phase synchronization and large-scale integration. Nat Rev Neurosci 2001;2:229–39.

133. Le Van Quyen M, Foucher J, Lachaux JP, et al. Comparison of Hilbert transform and wavelet methods for the analysis of neuronal synchrony. J Neurosci Meth 2001;111:83–98.

134. Andrzejak RG, Widman G, Lehnertz K, et al. The epileptic process as nonlinear deterministic dynamics in a stochastic environment – an evaluation of mesial temporal lobe epilepsy. Epilepsy Res 2001;44:129–40.

135. Slutzky MW, Cvitanovic P, Mogul DJ. Deterministic chaos and noise in three in vitro hippocampal models of epilepsy. Ann Biomed Eng 2001;29:1–12.

136. Worrell GA, Cranstoun SD, Echauz J, et al. Evidence for self-organized criticality in human epileptic hippocampus. Epilepsia 2002;43(S7):51.

137. Navaro V, Martinerie JM, Le Van Quyen M, et al. Seizure anticipation in human neocortical partial epilepsy. Brain 2002;125:640–55.

138. Osorio I, Frei MG, Giftakis J, et al. Performance reassessment of a real-time seizure-detection algorithm on long ECoG series. Epilepsia 2002; 43:1522–35.

139. Litt B, Lehnertz K. Seizure prediction and the pre-seizure period. Curr Opin Neurol 2002;15:173–7.

140. Litt B, Echauz J. Prediction of epileptic seizures. Lancet Neurology 2002;1:22–30.

141. D'Alessandro M, Vachtsevanos G, Lee HS, et al. A hybrid multifeature and multichannel analysis of continuous, prolonged intracranial EEG data for seizure prediction. Epilepsia 2002;43(S7):45.

142. Kalitzin S, Parra J, Velis DN, et al. Enhancement of phase clustering in the EEG/MEG gamma frequency band anticipates transitions to paroxysmal epileptiform activity in epileptic patients with known visual sensitivity. IEEE Trans Biomed Eng 2002;49:1279–86.

143. Quiroga RQ, Kraskov A, Kreuz T, et al. On the performance of different synchronization measures in real data: a case study on EEG signals. Phys Rev E 2002;65:041903.

144. Stam CJ, van Dijk BW. Synchronization likelihood: an unbiased measure of generalized synchronization in multivariate data sets. Physica D 2002;163: 236–51.

145. Netoff TI, Schiff SJ. Decreased neuronal synchronization during experimental seizures. J Neurosci 2002;22:7297–307.

146. Le Van Quyen M, Navaro V, Martinerie J, et al. Loss of phase synchrony in an animal model of partial status epilepticus. Epilepsia 2002;43(S7):17.

147. Mormann F, Kreuz T, Andrzejak RG, et al. Preictal state detection in continuous intracranial EEG recordings based on decreased phase synchronization: problems and pitfalls. Epilepsia 2002;43(S7):121.

148. Milton JG, Jung P, editors. Epilepsy as a dynamical disease. Heidelberg (Germany): Springer; 2003.

149. Chávez M, Le Van Quyen M, Navarro V, et al. Spatiotemporal dynamics prior to neocortical seizures: amplitude versus phase couplings. IEEE Trans Biomed Eng 2003;50:571–83.

150. D'Alessandro M, Esteller R, Vachtsevanos G, et al. Epileptic seizure prediction using hybrid feature selection over multiple intracranial EEG electrode contacts: a report of four patients. IEEE Trans Biomed Eng 2003;50:603–15.

151. De Clercq W, Lemmerling P, Van Huffel S, et al. Anticipation of epileptic seizures from standard EEG recordings. Lancet 2003;361:971.

152. Drury I, Smith B, Li D, et al. Seizure prediction using scalp electroencephalogram. Exp Neurol 2003;184:9–18.

153. Li D, Zhou W, Drury I, et al. Non-linear, non-invasive method for seizure anticipation in focal epilepsy. Math Biosci 2003;186:63–77.

154. Lopes da Silva F, Blanes W, Kalitzin S, et al. Epilepsies as a dynamical disease of brain systems: basic models of the transition between normal and epileptic activity. Epilepsia 2003;44:72–83.

155. Mormann F, Andrzejak RG, Kreuz T, et al. Automated detection of a pre-seizure state based on a decrease in synchronization in intracranial EEG recordings from epilepsy patients. Phys Rev E 2003;67:021912.

156. Mormann F, Kreuz T, Andrzejak RG, et al. Epileptic seizures are preceded by a decrease in synchronization. Epilepsy Res 2003;53:173–85.

157. Niederhauser JJ, Esteller R, Echauz J, et al. Detection of seizure precursors from depth-EEG using a sign periodogram transform. IEEE Trans Biomed Eng 2003;50:449–58.

158. Van Drongelen W, Nayak S, Frim DM, et al. Seizure anticipation in pediatric epilepsy: use of Kolmogorov entropy. Pediatr Neurol 2003;29:207–13.

159. Worrell GA, Parish L, Cranstoun SD, et al. High-frequency oscillations and seizure generation in neocortical epilepsy. Brain 2004;127(Pt 7): 1496–506.

160. Bartolomei F, Wendling F, Regis J, et al. Pre-ictal synchronicity in limbic networks of mesial temporal lobe epilepsy. Epilepsy Res 2004;61:89–104.

161. Cerf R, el-Ouasdad EH, Kahane P. Criticality and synchrony of fluctuations in rhythmical brain activity: pretransitional effects in epileptic patients. Biol Cybern 2004;90:239–55.

162. Gigola S, Ortiz F, D'Attellis CE, et al. Prediction of epileptic seizures using accumulated energy in a multiresolution framework. J Neurosci Methods 2004;138:107–11.

163. D'Alessandro M, Vachtsevanos G, Esteller R, et al. A multi-feature and multi-channel univariate

selection process for seizure prediction. Clin Neurophysiol 2005;116:506–16.

164. Esteller R, Echauz J, D'Alessandro M, et al. Continuous energy variation during the seizure cycle: towards an on-line accumulated energy. Clin Neurophysiol 2005;116:517–26.

165. Federico P, Abbott DF, Briellmann RS, et al. Functional MRI of the pre-ictal state. Brain 2005;128:1811–7.

166. Jouny CC, Franaszczuk PJ, Bergey GK. Signal complexity and synchrony of epileptic seizures: is there an identifiable preictal period? Clin Neurophysiol 2005;116:552–8.

167. Kalitzin S, Velis D, Suffczynski P, et al. Electrical brain stimulation paradigm for estimating the seizure onset site and the time to ictal transition in temporal lobe epilepsy. Clin Neurophysiol 2005; 116:718–28.

168. Le Van Quyen M, Soss J, Navarro V, et al. Preictal state identification by synchronization changes in long-term intracranial EEG recordings. Clin Neurophysiol 2005;116:559–68.

169. Mormann F, Kreuz T, Rieke C, et al. On the predictability of epileptic seizures. Clin Neurophysiol 2005; 116:569–87.

170. Navarro V, Martinerie J, Le Van Quyen M, et al. Seizure anticipation: do mathematical measures correlate with video-EEG evaluation? Epilepsia 2005;46:385–96.

171. Schiff SJ, Sauer T, Kumar R, et al. Neuronal spatiotemporal pattern discrimination: the dynamical evolution of seizure. Neuroimage 2005;28: 1043–55.

172. Percha B, Dzakpasu R, Parent J, et al. Transition from local to global phase synchrony in small world neural network and its possible implications for epilepsy. Phys Rev E 2005;72:031909.

173. Mormann F, Elger CE, Lehnertz K. Seizure anticipation: from algorithms to clinical practice [review]. Curr Opin Neurol 2006a;19:187–93.

174. Mormann F, Elger CE, Lehnertz K. Seizure anticipation: from algorithms to clinical practice. Curr Opin Neurol 2006;19(2):187–93.

175. Mormann F, Andrzejak RG, Elger CE, et al. Seizure prediction: the long and winding road. Brain 2007; 130(Pt 2):314–33.

176. Iasemidis LD. Synchronization in neural systems. Guest editorial for the special issue on synchronization in neural systems. Int J Neural Syst 2007; 17:1–2.

177. Chaovalitwongse W, Iasemidis LD, Sackellares JC, et al. Data mining in EEG: Application to epileptic brain disorders. In: Pardalos P, Boginski V, Vazacopoulos A, editors. Data mining in biomedicine. Springer series on optimization and its applications. New York: Springer; 2007. p. 459–82.

178. Feldt S, Osterhage H, Mormann F, et al. Inter- and intra-network communications during bursting

dynamics: applications to seizure prediction. Phys Rev E 2007;76:021920.

179. Schindler KA, Bialonski S, Horstmann MT, et al. Evolving functional network properties and synchronizability during human epileptic seizures. Chaos 2008;18:033119.

180. Lehnertz K. Epilepsy and nonlinear dynamics. J Biol Phys 2008;34(3):253–66.

181. Sackellares JC. Seizure prediction. Epilepsy Curr 2008;8:55–9.

182. Lehnertz K, Bialonski S, Horstmann MT, et al. Synchronization phenomena in human epileptic brain networks. J Neurosci Methods 2009;183:42–8.

183. Kuhnert MT, Elger CE, Lehnertz K. Long-term variability of global statistical properties of epileptic brain networks. Chaos 2010;20:043126.

184. McSharry PE, Smith LA, Tarassenko L. Prediction of epileptic seizures: are nonlinear methods relevant? Nat Med 2003;9:241–2.

185. Winterhalder M, Maiwald T, Voss HU, et al. The seizure prediction characteristic: a general framework to assess and compare seizure prediction methods. Epilepsy Behav 2003;4:318–25.

186. Shiau DS, Chaovalitwongse W, Iasemidis LD, et al. Nonlinear dynamical and statistical approaches to investigate dynamical transitions before epileptic seizures. In: Pardalos PM, Sackellares JC, Carney PR, et al, editors. Quantitative Neuroscience. Series on Biocomputing, vol. 2. Boston: Kluwer Academic Publishers; 2004. p. 239–49.

187. Kreuz T, Andrzejak RG, Mormann F, et al. Measure profile surrogates: a method to validate the performance of epileptic seizure prediction algorithms. Phys Rev E 2004;69:061915.

188. Maiwald T, Winterhalder M, Aschenbrenner-Scheibe R, et al. Comparison of three nonlinear seizure prediction methods by means of the seizure prediction characteristic. Physica D 2004;194: 357–68.

189. Pardalos PM, Chaovalitwongse W, Iasemidis LD, et al. Seizure warning algorithm based on optimization and nonlinear dynamics. J Math Program 2004;101:365–85.

190. Chaovalitwongse W, Iasemidis LD, Pardalos PM, et al. Performance of a seizure warning algorithm based on nonlinear dynamics of the intracranial EEG. Epilepsy Res 2005;64:93–113.

191. Iasemidis LD, Shiau DS, Pardalos PM, et al. Long-term prospective on-line real-time seizure prediction. J Clin Neurophysiol 2005;116: 532–44.

192. Chaovalitwongse W, Pardalos PM, Iasemidis LD, et al. Dynamical approaches and multi-quadratic integer programming for seizure prediction. Optimization Methods and Software 2005;20:383–94.

193. Iasemidis LD, Tsakalis K, Sackellares JC, et al. Comments on the inability of Lyapunov exponents

to predict epileptic seizures. Phys Rev Lett 2005; 94:019801.

194. Chaovalitwongse WA, Iasemidis LD, Pardalos PM, et al. Reply to comments by Mormann F, CE Elger, and Lehnertz K on the performance of a seizure warning algorithm based on the dynamics of intracranial EEG. Epilepsy Res 2006;72:85–7.

195. Chaovalitwongse WA, Iasemidis LD, Pardalos PM, et al. Reply to comments by M. Winterhalder, B. Schelter, A. Achulze-Bonhage and J. Timmer on the performance of a seizure warning algorithm based on the dynamics of intracranial EEG. Epilepsy Res 2006;72:82–4.

196. Winterhalder M, Schelter B, Maiwald T, et al. Spatio-temporal patient-individual assessment of synchronization changes for epileptic seizure prediction. J Clin Neurophysiol 2006;117: 2399–413.

197. Sackellares JC, Shiau DS, Principe JC, et al. Predictability analysis for an automated seizure prediction algorithm. J Clin Neurophysiol 2006;23: 509–20.

198. Kugiumtzis D, Papana A, Vlachos I, et al. Time series feature evaluation in discriminating preictal EEG states. Biological and Medical Data Analysis. Lecture Notes in Computer Science series 2006; 4345:298–310.

199. Schelter B, Winterhalder M, Maiwald T, et al. Testing statistical significance of multivariate time series analysis techniques for epileptic seizure prediction. Chaos 2006;16:013108.

200. Suffczynski P, Lopes da Silva FH, Parra J, et al. Dynamics of epileptic phenomena determined from statistics of ictal transitions. IEEE Trans Biomed Eng 2006;53:524–32.

201. Schelter B, Winterhalder M, Maiwald T, et al. Do false predictions of seizures depend on the state of vigilance? A report from two seizure prediction methods and proposed remedies. Epilepsia 2006; 7:2058–70.

202. Schelter B, Winterhalder M, Feldwisch genannt Drentrup H, et al. Seizure prediction: the impact of long prediction horizons. Epilepsy Res 2007; 73:213–7.

203. Kugiumtzis D, Vlachos I, Papana A, et al. Assessment of measures of scalar time series analysis in discriminating preictal states. Int J Bioelectromagn 2007;9(3):134–45.

204. Shiau DS, Iasemidis LD, Yang MCK, et al. Automated seizure prediction algorithm and its statistical assessment: a report from ten patients. In: Pardalos P, Boginski V, Vazacopoulos A, editors. Data mining in biomedicine. Springer series on optimization and its applications. Springer; 2007. p. 517–34.

205. Snyder DE, Echauz J, Grimes DB, et al. The statistics of a practical seizure warning system. J Neural Eng 2008;5(4):392–401.

206. Feldwisch-Drentrup H, Schelter B, Jachan M, et al. Joining the benefits: combining epileptic seizure prediction methods. Epilepsia 2010;51:1598.

207. Chisci L, Mavino A, Perferi G, et al. Real time epileptic seizure prediction using AR models and support vector machines. IEEE Trans. Biomed Eng 2010;57(5):1124–32.

208. Park Y, Luo L, Parhi KK, et al. Seizure prediction with spectral power of EEG using cost-sensitive support vector machines. Epilepsia 2011 [online].

209. Iasemidis LD, Tsakalis K, Osorio I, et al. Guest editorial for the special issue on "Neuromodulation and control of epileptic seizures". Int J Neural Syst 2009;19(3):v–vii.

210. Iasemidis LD, Schachter S, Worrell GA, et al. Guest editorial on "Neuromodulation in Epilepsy" Special Issue of Int J Neural Syst 2011;21:v–vi.

211. Yang XF, Schmidt BF, Rode DL, et al. Optical suppression of experimental seizures in rat brain slices. Epilepsia 2010;51(1):127–35.

212. Tsakalis K, Iasemidis LD. Prediction and control of epileptic seizures. International Conference and Summer School of Complexity in Science and Society, European Advanced Studies Conference V, Patras and Ancient Olympia, Greece, July 14–26, 2004.

213. Iasemidis LD, Sabesan S, Tsakalis K, et al. Prediction and control of epileptic seizures: The basis for brain pacemakers in epilepsy. 3rd European Medical and Biological Engineering Conference (EMBEC). Prague, November 20–25, 2005;11:6.

214. Shiau DS, Nair S, Iasemidis LD, et al. Seizure warning system and dynamic response to electrical stimulation in a rodent model of chronic limbic epilepsy. 3rd European Medical and Biological Engineering Conference (EMBEC). Prague, November 20–25, 2005;11:4.

215. Good L, Sabesan S, Iasemidis LD, et al. Real-time control of epileptic seizures. 3rd European Medical and Biological Engineering Conference (EMBEC). Prague, November 20–25, 2005;11:6.

216. Tsakalis K, Chakravarthy N, Iasemidis LD. Theoretical concepts of control with applications to epilepsy. 3rd European Medical and Biological Engineering Conference (EMBEC). Prague, November 20–25, 2005;11:6.

217. Tsakalis K, Chakravarthy N, Iasemidis LD. Control of epileptic seizures: models of chaotic oscillator networks. Joint 44th IEEE Conference on Decision and Control and the European Control Conference (CDC-ECC'05). Seville, December 12–15, 2005:2975–81.

218. Suffczynski P, Lopes da Silva F, Parra J, et al. Epileptic transitions: model predictions and experimental validation. J Clin Neurophysiol 2005; 22:288–99.

219. Tsakalis K, Chakravarthy N, Sabesan S, et al. A feedback control systems view of epileptic seizures. Cybernetics Syst Anal 2006;42:483–95.

220. Tsakalis K, Iasemidis LD. Control aspects of a theoretical model for epileptic seizures. Int J Bifurcat Chaos 2006;16:2013–27.

221. Chakravarthy N, Sabesan S, Iasemidis LD, et al. Modeling and controlling synchronization in a neuron-level population model. Int J Neural Syst 2007;17:123–38.

222. Chakravarthy N, Sabesan S, Spanias A, et al. A feedback systems approach to modeling neural firing-rate homeostasis. 46th IEEE Conference on Decision and Control (CDC). New Orleans (LA), December 12–14, 2007. Avaliable at: http://ieeexplore.ieee.org/xpl/mostRecentIssue.jsp?punumber=4433999(IEEE press).

223. Suffczynski P, Kalitzin S, Lopes da Silva FH, et al. Active paradigms of seizure anticipation – a computer model evidence for necessity of stimulation. Phys Rev E 2008;78:051917.

224. Iasemidis LD, Sabesan S, Good LB, et al. Closed-loop control of epileptic seizures via deep brain stimulation in a rodent model of chronic epilepsy. World Congress on Medical Physics and Biomedical Engineering 2009: 7–12.

225. Iasemidis LD, Sabesan S, Chakravarthy N, et al. Brain dynamics and modeling in epilepsy: prediction and control studies. In: Dana SK, Roy PK, Kurths J, editors. Complex dynamics of physiological systems: from heart to brain. Springer series on complexity. Dordrecht (The Netherlands): Springer-Verlag; 2009. p. 185–214.

226. Chakravarthy N, Tsakalis K, Sabesan S, et al. Homeostasis of brain dynamics in epilepsy: a feedback control systems perspective of seizures. Ann Biomed Eng 2009;37:565–85.

227. Chakravarthy N, Sabesan S, Iasemidis LD, et al. Controlling epileptic seizures in a neural mass model. J Comb Optim 2009;17:98–116.

228. Good L, Sabesan S, Marsh S, et al. Control of synchronization of brain dynamics leads to control of epileptic seizures in rodents. Int J Neural Syst 2009;19(3):173–96.

229. Sabesan S, Narayanan K, Prasad A, et al. Information flow in coupled nonlinear systems: application to the epileptic human brain. In: Pardalos P, Boginski V, Vazacopoulos A, editors. Data mining in biomedicine. Springer series on optimization and its applications. Springer; 2007. p. 483–504.

230. Sabesan S, Good L, Tsakalis K, et al. Information flow and application to epileptogenic focus localization from EEG. IEEE Trans Neural Syst Rehabil Eng 2009;17(3):244–53.

231. Iasemidis LD, Sabesan S, Good L, et al. A new look into epilepsy as a dynamical disorder: seizure prediction, resetting and control. In: Schwartzkroin P, editor. Encyclopedia of Basic Epilepsy Research. Oxford: Academic Press; 2009. p. 1295–302.

Features and Futures: Seizure Detection in Partial Epilepsies

Yu Han, MS[a], Yue-Loong Hsin, MD[b], Tomor Harnod, MD, PhD[c], Wentai Liu, PhD[a],*

KEYWORDS

- Ictal EEG • Intracranial EEG
- Independent component analysis • Partial epilepsy
- Seizure detection

Many factors underlying basic epileptic conditions determine the characteristics of epileptic seizures and the therapeutic outcome. Diagnosis and treatment rely on the clinical manifestations as well as electroencephalographic (EEG) epileptic activities. Any EEG abnormality will increase the recurrence risk and indicate drug therapy in cases that are unprovoked.[1,2] Ictal symptoms, which correlate with seizure EEG activity, can guide neurosurgeons on epilepsy surgery. Modern neuroengineers use engineering technology to analyze EEG signals in investigating and treating epilepsy. For example, a pivotal trial that used responsive brain neurostimulation (RNS System, NeuroPace, Inc, Mountain View, CA) achieved positive results by significantly reducing the frequency of seizures for epileptic patients with medical intractability.[3,4] From the pathophysiologic point of view, it is feasible to achieve automatic detection of epileptic neurophysiology using an implanted device, and to concomitantly reset brain dynamics from the ictal to the interictal state by electrical stimulation over specific brain regions. However, to improve and strengthen the effectiveness of current treatments, more accurate detection of seizure activity over time and delineation of epileptogenic regions are critical for on-demand therapy.

In the early 1970s, Viglione and Walsh[5] preceded seizure prediction by using linear analysis approaches to extract seizure precursors from surface EEG recordings of absence seizures. Thereafter, many algorithms were developed to quantify EEG or intracranial EEG for seizure prediction or detection. With the advent of the physical-mathematical theory, the fusion of sophisticated techniques based on nonlinear dynamic systems is superior to those based on linear analyses in dealing with the changes in complexity or energy preictally. However, the performance validation of nonlinear systems is still not statistically significant, and the present-day systems are still not practical enough to be embedded in the implantable devices that warn of impending seizures or trigger therapeutic impulse responsively. While many investigators focus on improving mathematics for seizure prediction rather than on realizing the pathophysiology of epileptogenesis, the performance of the current seizure-detection algorithms is not satisfactory. There is no doubt that improvement in performance can be obtained once the algorithm more closely refers to the underlying mechanisms.

This article briefly reviews the fundamentals of the EEG, interictal, and ictal electrical activities of both

The authors have nothing to disclose.

[a] Department of Electrical Engineering, University of California Santa Cruz, 1156 High Street, Santa Cruz, CA 95064, USA

[b] Department of Neurology, Hualien Tzu Chi Medical Center, No. 707, Sec.3, Chung Yang Road, Hualein 970, Taiwan

[c] Department of Neurosurgery, Hualein Tzu Chi Medical Center, No. 707, Sec.3, Chung Yang Road, Hualein 970, Taiwan

* Corresponding author.

E-mail address: wentai@soe.ucsc.edu

extracranial and intracranial EEG of partial epilepsies, based on the information obtained from epilepsy patients who have undergone epilepsy surgery. The authors also present the status of their current research, focusing on decomposed seizure sources and the rendered spatial-temporal transitions in focal seizure.

GENERATION OF BRAINWAVES

The neuronal networks that generate brainwaves and subcorticocortical loops are modeled to explain the rhythms of superficial field potentials. The near-surface apical dendrites of pyramidal neurons are primarily responsible for summating the afferent impulses into postsynaptic potentials and forming effective dipoles. The recording of the field potentials shows sinusoidal fluctuations when there is a periodic sequence of the afferent bursts.[6] Once populations of neurons are synchronously activated as in the definition of epileptic activity, the activity can be recorded as a convolution of the unit dipoles. This convolved activity may also be represented as a dipole or sheet of dipoles along the cortex. The theory of brainwave formation thus supports the application of independent component analysis, which is discussed in the later section of this article.

FEATURES OF EPILEPTIC BRAINWAVES

Since Frederic Gibbs started to use EEG to assess epilepsy, EEG has revolutionized the field of epileptology. Many EEG abnormalities including spikes, sharp waves, spike-and-slow-wave complexes, polyspikes, and hypsarrhythmia are interpreted as epileptic activities. In the widely used classification of epileptic seizures proposed by the Commission on Classification and Terminology (1981), EEG features have become an integral part.[7] By definition, partial seizures or generalized seizures are those in which the first clinical changes indicate that the initial involvement starts at the unilateral or bilateral hemisphere. Clinicians usually cannot determine the types of epileptic seizures or syndrome when the clinical data are inadequate or incomplete, therefore the initial EEG might support the differentiation.

Electroencephalographic Features of Generalized Seizures

The generalized seizure types include absence, myoclonic, clonic, tonic, tonic-clonic, and atonic seizure. Regular and symmetric spike-and-slow-wave complexes at 3 Hz are easily recognized as the ictal EEG of typical absence seizures. The polyspike-and-slow-wave, spike-and-slow-wave, or sharp-and-slow-wave complexes concurrently appearing at brief shocklike contraction confined to the face, trunk, or extremities, support the myoclonic seizure diagnosis. A sudden lapse of muscle tone occurrence leading to a head drop or a slump, polyspikes-and-slow-wave, or flattening or low-voltage fast activity can also be found simultaneously. Usually known as grand mal, tonic-clonic seizures are the most frequently encountered of the generalized seizure type. The grand mal attack is initiated by an abrupt loss of voltage of a few seconds' duration; there is evidence of very fast (20–40/s) activity in all leads. After the first transition phase of seizure onset, rhythmic activity at about 10 per second with rapidly increasing amplitude dominates the EEG. Subsequently the initial fast activity enters the theta range, followed by repetitive bursts of spikes during the clonic phase. All of the epileptiform discharges in different generalized seizures can be displayed on the interictal scalp EEG independently.

Electroencephalographic Features of Partial Seizures

As clinical features, the variety of the ictal EEG of partial seizures is remarkable. From the clinical perspective, partial seizure attacks may be undetermined because either the presence of change in mental status and inappropriate behaviors from focal epilepticus of frontal lobe origin, or the presence of visceral ictal symptoms from temporal lobe origin, is not easily noticed. Hence, epileptologists may not be able to identify the ictal EEGs if the subtle onsets on the EEG display are not carefully examined when reading the records from patients with partial epilepsies. From the EEG perspective, in the case of temporal lobe epilepsy the interictal scalp EEG may show no abnormality, slight asymmetry of the background activity, or even bilateral temporal spikes.

The initial ictal EEG change of temporal lobe seizure may consist of clear spikes, but often only theta activity is seen. In the early work of Gibbs and colleagues[8] and Gibbs and Gibbs,[9] the ictal EEG activity of the psychomotor seizure was described as a special type of seizure discharge characterized by bursts of serrated slow waves, 4 flat-topped waves per second, and 6 high-voltage rhythmic activity per second (**Fig. 1**). Many investigators including Gastaut, Vigouroux, and Klass emphasized the variability of the ictal EEG.

To localize the ictal foci in patients with partial seizures of frontal origin is much more difficult than for patients with seizures of temporal lobe origin, although the ictal EEG patterns are still found to consist of fast-activity mixed spikes,

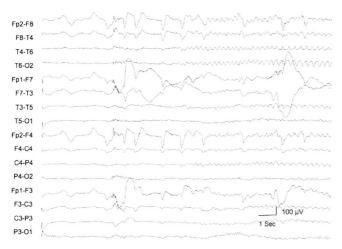

Fig. 1. Temporal lobe epilepsy in a 30-year-old man with discontinuation of ongoing movement and dystonic posturing of right limbs at seizure onset. Ictal EEG at seizure onset: repetitive focal sharp waves over the right temporal region at 4 Hz.

rhythmic spikes, rhythmic spike-and-wave complexes, or rhythmic slow waves. Because of the inaccessibility of foci on the mesial and orbital aspects of the frontal lobes and the rapid propagation and easy generalization, only approximately 30% of frontal lobe complex partial seizures are accompanied by some type of localizing EEG finding (**Fig. 2**).

Seizures emanating from the parietal or occipital lobes are mainly "simple" without impairment of consciousness. Subjective symptoms such as somatic illusion or elementary visual hallucinations with correlated interictal EEG abnormality help differential diagnosis (**Fig. 3**).

Intracranial Electroencephalographic Features of Partial Seizures

Historically, Berger was the first person to perform intraoperative EEG with electrodes placed over the dural surface in patients with skull defects. In the early 1950s, Penfield and Erickson[10] directly recorded electrical activity from the exposed cortex during surgical procedures. These investigators recognized the large amplitude and short duration of clear spike discharges that occurred as single sporadic spikes, groups of spikes in short bursts, or in the form of a multiple-spike discharge, and in some cases as a spike and slow-wave

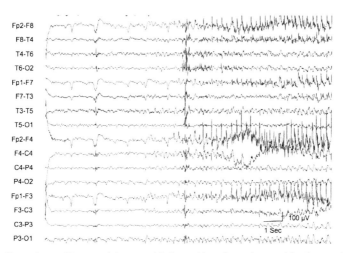

Fig. 2. Frontal lobe epilepsy in an 18-year-old man with forced head-turning and body rotation at seizure onset. Ictal EEG at seizure onset: repetitive large-voltage sharp waves separated by small-voltage fast activity toward the frontal regions with maximum at the right frontal lobe.

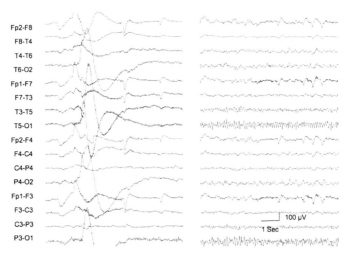

Fig. 3. Occipital lobe epilepsy in a 26-year-old man with visual hallucination and eye deviation at seizure onset. Ictal EEG at seizure onset (*left*): small spiky alpha activity at 10 Hz after a large-amplitude delta wave over the left occipital lobe at seizure onset. Ictal EEG 10 seconds later (*right*): ictal activity transited into sharp contoured theta activity at 7 Hz.

complex. The "interictal" cortical potentials expressed by "acute" electrocorticography (ECoG) objectively identified epileptogenic lesions. These zones would then be surgically removed from the cortex.

The improvement of "chronic" intracranial implantation of strip-electrodes and grid electrodes greatly facilitates the recognition of the pre-ictal and ictal electrical activities. At present, a typical ictal ECoG could be characterized with (1) initially fast activity with low amplitude in a few channels and then propagating to neighboring channels; (2) activity that slows down with gaining amplitude; (3) lateral bursting of high-voltage poly-spike and slow waves separated by prolonging suppressed activity before seizure termination (**Fig. 4**). Aside from the difference in large voltage (cortical EEG activity exceeding 500 μV), essentially the morphology of interictal epileptiform discharges such as spikes, sharp waves, and spike-and-slow-wave complexes is very similar to the conventional scalp EEG. The signals of intracranial EEG are rarely obscured by muscular and environmental artifacts.

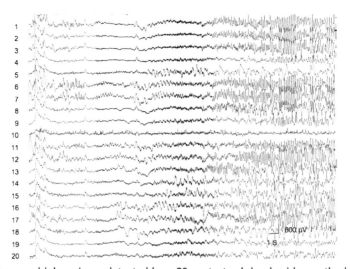

Fig. 4. Left lateral temporal lobe seizure detected by a 20-contact subdural grid over the left temporal gyri. A diffuse attenuation of background activity at seizure onset followed by small-amplitude fast activity at some channels, then followed by wild spread of large-amplitude sharp waves.

SCATTERED NATURE OF SEIZURE FOCI

There is increasing experimental evidence that an epileptic region of the brain more likely consists of multiple small distributed hyperexcitable networks. Schevon and colleagues[11] obtained recordings from 5 patients with microelectrode arrays positioned within the boundaries of an intracranial grid. These investigators observed different types of rhythmic electrical activity without any clinical manifestation, and defined microdischarges as localized epileptiform discharges appearing on one or a few adjacent recording electrodes. The microdischarges that occurred in repetitive and evolving patterns were defined as microseizures. The microseizures have complicated the analyses of seizure spatiotemporal dynamics, and have unmasked the unreliability of previous methods for seizure detection.[12]

EPILEPTIC SEIZURE DETECTION

Monitoring epileptic activity and detecting seizure onset are important issues in neurophysiology, because prompt therapeutic intervention could thus be enabled to prevent epileptic patients with medical intractable partial epilepsies from getting injured or to suppress the ongoing ictal activities. Starting in the 1970s, several attempts have been made to monitor seizure activity. Ives and colleagues[13] reported a triggered EEG system that was designed to passively record EEG once a seizure occurred. This system was limited to recording seizures that were accompanied by clinical manifestations, whereas seizures with no clinical behavior but with electrographic demonstrations were missed. This shortcoming motivated the development of automatic seizure-detection systems in the next few decades.

Rule-Based EEG Feature Recognition

Gotman,[14] one of the pioneer investigators addressing the issue of automated seizure-pattern recognition, reported an effective seizure-detection method in 1982. This method, by choosing the relative amplitude, average duration, and coefficient of duration variation of elementary halfwaves as the criteria of detection, suffered from high false positives (FPs) caused by nonepileptiform bursts and inevitable artifacts. In 1990 this algorithm was further improved, whereby the criterion of average relative amplitude was relaxed and an extra epoch was incorporated into the background, targeted at reducing both missed and false detections.[15] Although approximate three-quarter seizures could be automatically detected (on 293 recordings from 49 patients), a high FP

rate still remained. In 1997, Qu and Gotman[16,17] reported an interesting early seizure warning system with an excellent onset detection rate and with an average delay of 9.35 seconds after onset. The individualized system used a nearest-neighbor classifier incorporating patient-specific information to achieve both high detection rate and low FP rate. The results looked attractive; however, this method was restricted to detecting seizures that were similar to template patterns used in classifier training stage. Therefore, some kinds of seizures with different generation mechanisms and evolutions may not be recognized by this system.

Since the 1990s there have been numerous reports describing various rule-based methods to detect seizure activity by either time or frequency domain techniques.[18–21] Murro and colleagues[18] used 3 quantified EEG features, namely, dominant frequency, relative power, and rhythmicity, to differentiate seizure from nonseizure activities for the ECoGs of 8 patients. Harding[19] designed an automated seizure-monitoring system for patients with indwelling recording electrodes to trace both the amplitude and frequency of spikes. A seizure event was declared when the count of large magnitude of the sample-to-sample differences (MDV) in a 5-second epoch exceeded the channel-specific thresholds. The system performance had 86% detection accuracy, with 1.26 brief spike bursts and 0.67 artifacts per hour. In 1998, Osorio and colleagues[20] reported a real-time detector with 100% detection sensitivity and zero FP rate tested with ECoG data containing 125 seizures and 205 nonseizures from 16 subjects. A defined quantitative energy measure, called "seizure intensity," was calculated from signals after wavelet-based filtering and sequential median filtering. The same data were used for both parameter optimization and algorithm validation. More testing results using off-line ECoGs were reported in 2002.[21] All clinical seizures were detected, while some of undetected subclinical and unclassified seizures could be captured when using an adaptation technique. The FP rate was restricted to as low as less than 4 per day.

Training-Based Artificial Neural Network for Seizure Detection

Since the 1990s, there has been a growing interest in using an artificial neural network (ANN)[22] as an alternative nonlinear analysis tool for epileptiform activity detection.[23–27] The advantage of ANN-based detection lies in its ability to learn by any training features defined by rule makers, making it possible to make a decision based on the classification of such features. Because a training process is of particular necessity and importance for such methods, the performance, to a great degree, depends on the training data and extracted features. Pradhan and colleagues[23] used ANN for detecting interictal epileptiform discharges (EDs) by using one patient's EEG for training and another 4 patients' data for algorithm testing. The reported specificity and sensitivity of ED echo detection were 74.8% and 67%. Weng and Khorasani[24] demonstrated an improved adaptive structure neural network to automate recognition of epileptic seizures in EEG. Five epileptic features, the same as those proposed by Qu and Gotman,[16,17] were extracted. To reduce the FP rate, nonseizure patterns closer to the boundary of seizure patterns were selected for training, which unfortunately deteriorated the detection accuracy. Webber and colleagues[25] developed an EEG seizure detector using 31 time-frequency features as the input to an ANN to classify the EEG into several patterns: artifacts, for example, muscle and chewing noise, and normal patterns as well as seizure activity. Results from 78 selected files not included in the training procedure gave the detection rate of 76% and FP rate of 1.0/h. As the investigators mentioned, the number of features to be trained in this method could be reduced, because some were highly correlated and redundant information was involved. Gabor and colleagues[26] used a self-organizing map (SOM) network to generalize spectral features of 98 training seizures from 30 patients into 6 categories. A training pattern matched wavelet filter was used before seizure detection to reduce false detections. Rule-based criteria, such as the relative amplitude, number of matching nodes, and so forth, were used in detections that could be potentially patient specific to obtain better performance. The results from 24 records tested from 22 patients showed that a 90% detection rate with 0.71/h FP rate was achievable. A follow-up report improved this algorithm by increasing the training examples from 98 to 109 and the number of network nodes from 6 to 7.[27] The improved algorithm was validated with 200 records from 65 patients, and the reported seizure-detection rate was 92.8% while the mean FP rate was 1.35/h. This method required several empirical detection parameters to be well defined, and prior tuning of parameters may be needed to achieve the best performance.

It should be noted that because in principle the ANN-based method relies on the extracted features for training, the detection performance could inevitably be affected by artifacts, and the relative high FP rate might be unavoidable. On the other hand, if some data was chosen for both training and testing, the reported detection accuracy may be higher than that in the real case.

Other techniques that target epileptic seizure detection have been reported, such as the support vector machine,[28] wavelet-based feature extraction,[29,30] and independent component analysis (ICA).[31–33] Other investigators[34,35] discuss the important issue of neonatal epileptic seizure monitoring and detection, because the clinical manifestations of newborns are usually subtle.

INDEPENDENT COMPONENT ANALYSIS

ICA has become a powerful tool in solving blind source separation (BSS) problems.[36–38] The main objective of ICA is to extract the underlying independent components (ICs) from their measured mixtures with the only assumptions being that the components are mutually statistically independent and the instantaneous mixing process is linear. The most apparent advantages of this technique include there being no requirement for prior knowledge regarding the sources to be extracted, unlike for the adaptive filtering technique, and that both the ICs and mixing process can be recovered during the decomposition procedure.

In the past few years ICA has been introduced into the study of neurophysiology, such as for event-related potential (ERP) studies,[39,40] EEG signal analysis,[31–33,41] and artifact removal.[42–46] For the EEG or ECoG signals of epileptic patients, seizure activity can be considered independent of the superimposed artifacts and the background normal brain activity. Therefore, with artifact immunity, ICA would facilitate feature extraction and classification of epileptic seizure activity as well as epileptogenic source localization in the analysis of EEG/ECoG signals. Motivated by this reason, recently some researchers have begun to make attempts on incorporating this powerful technique into seizure-activity analysis. Nam and colleagues[31] applied ICA to 24 ictal scalp EEGs from 14 patients with medial temporal lobe epilepsy (TLE). One to 3 ictal components per patient were visually identified according to the morphologic characteristics of rhythmic theta waves. Selective reconstruction was then performed by choosing 3 components with the largest 2- to 10-Hz power in order to omit the eye-movement and muscle-movement artifacts. However, the epileptic components were not recognized in an automated way, and some seizure-involved brain activities with frequencies larger than 10 Hz, such as alpha and beta waves, were excluded in the EEG reconstruction. Hoeve and colleagues[32] used the change of absolute sum, calculated in each row of the estimated mixing matrix, as an indicator for detecting paroxysmal activity. Using scalp EEG recordings of 5 patients, the reported sensitivity and selectivity were 74% and 19%, respectively, which implied a reasonably high FP rate. In fact the chosen indicator, which measured the projection effect of all decomposed components on each channel, did not take into account the massive information of the components (perhaps not the epileptic ones) themselves. For this reason, high false detections may not have been avoided because true ictal activity was not well differentiated from the artifacts. In addition, topographic mapping of seizure sources onto the electrode surface was not investigated in this study. Subasi and Gursoy[33] decomposed EEGs into sub-bands using discrete wavelet transform and extracted statistical features from those sub-bands. ICA was selected as 1 of 3 approaches for feature dimension reduction to facilitate seizure differentiation of support vector machine classifier. Impressive results with ICA (nearly 100%) were demonstrated for both sensitivity and specificity. However, no individual ictal component was detected and spatial relations of seizure-source mapping were not analyzed either. This method is computational intensive and is not practical for real-time seizure detection.

Originating from different decomposition criteria or constraints, ICA can be classified into several categories along with its development, such as FastICA,[47,48] Infomax ICA,[41,49] topographic ICA (TICA),[50,51] constrained ICA (CICA),[52–54] and multidimensional ICA.[55] Among such ICA algorithms, the FastICA approach was selected in this study for 3 reasons. First, the FastICA has fast convergence (at least quadratic[48]) and is computationally simple, which allows for potential online implementation for seizure detection in epilepsy monitoring. Second, prior knowledge about the morphology and the distribution of the underlying sources is not needed. This advantage accommodates various morphologies of seizure patterns and limited available knowledge about the generation mechanism of epilepsy. Finally, compared with Infomax ICA, the number of components is not determined before the iteration procedure begins for FastICA. In fact it is extremely difficult to estimate the number of independent seizure and nonseizure sources from multichannel EEGs or ECoGs. Therefore, finding all the potential sources can be regarded as a more reasonable option to capture the seizure activity.

PROPOSED SEIZURE-DETECTION METHOD

This section describes an ICA-based epileptic seizure-detection method using multichannel ECoG signals. This method is illustrated in **Fig. 5**, and currently the detection procedure is working off-line. In this method, a preprocessing procedure is firstly conducted on the recorded data in each epoch to simplify and condition well the subsequent decomposition procedures. The mean of the data is removed and the data are whitened using eigenvalue analysis. The FastICA algorithm is then used on the preprocessed data to iteratively uncover each IC and at the same time to estimate the mixing matrix that has mapped the underlying ICs to recorded signals. To obtain the frequency-domain representation of each IC, fast Fourier transform (FFT) is applied to each component. From the spectra of all the uncovered ICs, several useful features of the recording data can be extracted. In this study, the authors choose the spectrum power at an empirically defined frequency band (eg, 5–20 Hz), and the frequencies with the largest and the second largest amplitudes in the whole frequency band, as 3 critical features.

The detection of epileptic seizure activity, when viewed as a special event, can be treated as a statistical hypothesis test, whereby null hypothesis (H_0) is no seizure in the epoch whereas alternative hypothesis (H_1) marks the event of a seizure happening. To make a decision as to whether seizure occurs, two major criteria are combined to assure that ICs with fast and strong rhythmic activities are identifiable as seizure components: (1) the calculated spectrum power is higher than a predefined threshold, which is determined by the sampling frequency, bandwidth of interest, the number of points in FFT, and a power scaling factor; and (2) the frequency with the largest amplitude or the second largest amplitude locates within the interested band as previously defined. The second criterion is added to the critical region because it is shown to effectively reduce false detections caused by short paroxysmal activity with large low-frequency power. The criterion-based detection procedure is conducted on each

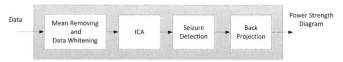

Fig. 5. Detection method for ICA-based epileptic seizure.

IC sequentially to decide whether it is epileptiform or not. If one or more ICs satisfy the detection criteria, the null hypothesis is declared to be rejected and the event of seizure activity may occur. Those ICs will be labeled as seizure ICs, and a reduced mixing matrix can be obtained by removing the columns of the estimated mixing matrix that correspond to the nonseizure ICs.

To investigate the effects of seizure ICs on recording electrodes, a back projection is further performed by multiplying the reduced mixing matrix with the identified seizure ICs. A power-strength diagram, which plots the power strength of each channel after back projection, can be used to highlight the seizure-associated channels. Thus the channels with relative larger power are regarded to be much more involved with the detected seizure sources.

RESULTS USING PROPOSED SEIZURE-DETECTION METHOD

This section shows some preliminary results of the authors' proposed epileptic seizure-detection method using ECoG recordings of epileptic patients. As an example, an ictal recording with a 4 × 5 electrode grid recorded from one patient suffering from partial TLE was firstly used to illustrate the whole detection procedure. This recording has 71,000 samples, approximately equivalent to 4.6 minutes at the sampling rate of 256 Hz. An epoch containing 4096 samples (16 seconds) was chosen as a base unit for ICA process and seizure detection. This moderate length, avoiding both longer detection latency

and less informative data collection, would facilitate the FFT operation in spectrum analysis.

The ictal ECoG waveforms of all channels in a selected epoch are shown in **Fig. 6**. By applying the FastICA algorithm, 20 decomposed ICs were extracted sequentially from the original signals, as shown in **Fig. 7**. **Fig. 8** presents the spectra of these ICs after using FFT on each IC. Carefully reviewing these spectrum plots, one can see that a group of ICs expresses a different spectral property than the other ICs: it has a relatively higher power in the interested frequency band compared with the power in other frequencies. Thus in the context of seizure detection, spectral features may be informative as a signature for epileptic activity. Based on the proposed detection criteria, 8 ICs were identified as potential seizure sources: IC4, IC5, IC7, IC10, IC11, IC16, IC17, and IC19. **Fig. 9**A shows the power-strength diagram on the electrode array after back projection by incorporating only epileptic components. Compared with **Fig. 9**B showing power strengths of the original ECoG data, the strengths of channels with normal activity but strongly interfered with artifacts, for example, channels C5 to C8, were suppressed, and the channels highly involved by epileptic seizures stand out, such as C12, C13, and C17. These results agree with the visual inspection on the ECoG waveforms by epileptologists, and to some extent confirm the correctness of the independent source decomposition and back-projection procedures. Because of the ability to explicitly reflect seizure-affected channels, a power-strength diagram would be a less labor-intensive indication for epileptologists performing

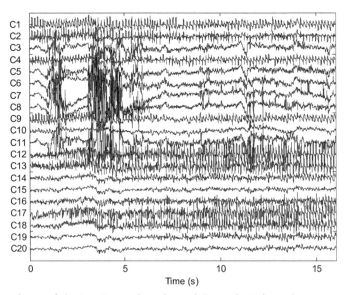

Fig. 6. Ictal ECoG waveforms of the 4 × 5 recording channels in a selected epoch.

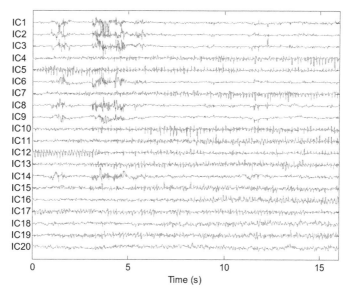

Fig. 7. Waveforms of decomposed ICs.

epilepsy diagnosis than the traditional review of a series of waveforms on ECoGs of epileptic patients.

Further, **Fig. 10** demonstrates how the power strengths of 20 channels vary with time using the same ECoG recording, so as to give a rough idea on the detection accuracy of this method in terms of seizure-onset time and involved channels. The waveforms of the recording were visually scored by one epileptologist separately before the analysis was performed, and the electrographic onset (EO) was marked (EO = 120.7 seconds in this recording). Because all the 16-second samples in each epoch have to be ready to calculate the

power strength for a time instant, the time axis in **Fig. 10** ranges from 16 seconds to the end of this recording. Moving epochs were used to improve the resolution of the power-strength diagram, with 256 samples (1 second) as each moving step. The power-strength diagram of the original ECoG data is shown in **Fig. 10**A, where the black arrow indicates the EO as a reference and the blue dotted arrow indicates the selected epoch of the aforementioned example. It was found that most channels expressed higher power strengths after seizure occurred. However, after performing ICA, seizure detection, and back projection on the data, the seizure-involved channels highlighted in

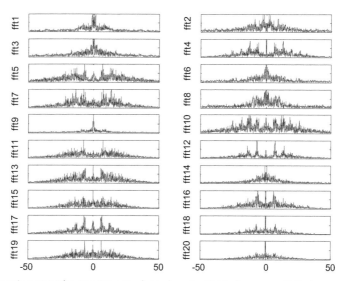

Fig. 8. Spectra of ICs using FFT. The spectra are plotted up to 50 Hz for an explicit demonstration.

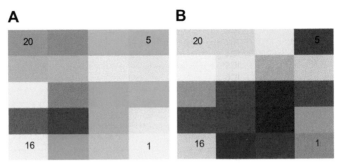

Fig. 9. Power-strength diagram of recording electrode grid. The numbers 1 to 20 indicate channels corresp‹ to those shown in ECoG waveforms. (*A*) Power strengths of signals after back projection; (*B*) power stren‹ the original ECoG data.

Fig. 10B, showing that the power strengths start to change immediately after EO. The detection latency equals approximately one epoch duration. Because the data are analyzed in the off-line manner, it is not easy to obtain the "true" latency with respect to EO. The latency should include an additional latency, because of the computational time required for seizure-activity detection. However, with the rapid advancement of computer technology, this amount of latency might be too small to be worthy of inclusion. Thus the epoch duration, as one of the important parameters in this method, becomes the dominant factor in determining the "true" detection latency. Due to space limitations, this article does not address the criteria for selection of parameters.

The proposed seizure-detection algorithm has been tested by applying 24 ictal ECoGs from 13 patients available at Hualein Tzu Chi Medical Center, Taiwan. All seizures were captured and

ictal-related channels were identified, have been verified by epileptologists. F‹ more, this algorithm has also been tested both ictal and interictal ECoG data re‹ from 21 patients at the Epilepsy Center University Hospital of Freiburg, Germany. ictal recordings containing 87 seizures a‹ interictal recordings of approximately 504 long were used to test the statistical perfor‹ of the proposed method. The results the sensitivity and specificity to be 6‹ and 96.35%, respectively, with 16-second detection. For this test, the reported sensi‹ not so high because 18 seizures from 4 p‹ are classified as short seizures, the dura‹ which is much less than 16 seconds‹ exceeding the detection precision requi‹ for a 16-second epoch length. After sho‹ the epoch length to 4 seconds, a sensit‹ 91.95% is achieved.

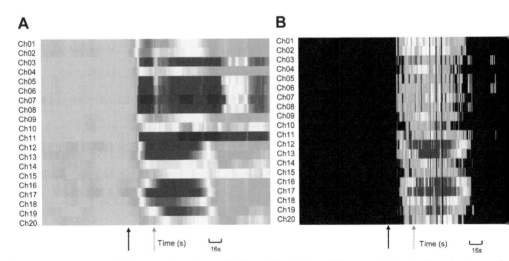

Fig. 10. Power-strength diagram changing with time. The black solid arrow indicates the electrograph‹ marked separately by one epileptologist, and the blue dotted arrow indicates the tested epoch of the e‹ shown in **Fig. 9.** (*A*) Power strengths of the original ECoG data; (*B*) power strengths of signals aft‹ projection.

SUMMARY

As one of the most serious neurologic disorders, epilepsy affects nearly 1% of the population worldwide. Timely therapeutic intervention for patients undergoing clinical seizures requires a seizure-monitoring system able to perform epileptic seizure detection with both high sensitivity and high specificity. For those patients with intractable seizures, surgical treatment is of necessity, whereby precise epileptogenic zone identification is required to effectively perform the final resection. ICA, a powerful tool for extraction of epileptic sources from the measurements, provides a new perspective for examining the issues of epileptic seizure detection and epileptogenic source localization. This article presents the authors' current research on the ICA-based seizure-detection approach, following discussions on mechanisms and features of brainwaves and the new concept of microseizures. Experimental results show high detection accuracy with high specificity, which encourages the authors to conduct further research on seizure dynamics and evolution, and to study the important issue of source positioning in the future.

ACKNOWLEDGMENTS

This work is partially supported by an endowment fund from the Human Signal Engine (HSE) LLC for the Chan Soon-Shiung Bionic Engineering Center at the University of California at Santa Cruz from Human Signal Engine (HSE).

REFERENCES

1. Schreiner A, Pohlmann-Eden B. Value of the early electroencephalogram after a first unprovoked seizure. Clin Electroencephalogr 2003;34(3):140–4.
2. Wirrell EC. Prognostic significance of interictal epileptiform discharges in newly diagnosed seizure disorders. J Clin Neurophysiol 2010;27(4):239–48.
3. Echauz J, Esteller R, Tcheng T, et al. Long-term validation of detection algorithms suitable for an implantable device. In: Annual Meeting of the American Epilepsy Society (AES). Philadelphia, November 30–December 5, 2001.
4. Morrell MJ, Hirsch LJ, Bergey G, et al. Long-term safety and efficacy of the RNS system in adults with medically intractable partial onset seizures. In: Annual Meeting of the American Epilepsy Society (AES). Seattle, December 5–9, 2008.
5. Viglione SS, Walsh GO. Proceedings: epileptic seizure prediction. Electroencephalogr Clin Neurophysiol 1975;39(4):435–6.
6. Speckmann EJ, Elger CE, Altrup U. Neurophysiologic basis of the electroencephalogram. In: Wyllie E, editor. The Treatment of Epilepsy: Principles & Practice. Philadelphia: Lippincott Williams & Wilkins; 2006. p. 127–39.
7. Proposal for revised clinical and electroencephalographic classification of epileptic seizures. From the Commission on Classification and Terminology of the International League Against Epilepsy. Epilepsia 1981;22(4):489–501.
8. Gibbs FA, Gibbs EL, Lennox WG. Epilepsy: a paroxysmal cerebral dysrhythmia. Epilepsy Behav 2002; 3(4):395–401.
9. Gibbs FA, Gibbs EL. Atlas of electroencephalography. Cambridge (MA): Addison-Wesley; 1952.
10. Penfield W, Erickson TC. Epilepsy and cerebral localization. Springfield (IL): Charles C. Thomas; 1941.
11. Schevon CA, Ng SK, Cappell J, et al. Microphysiology of epileptiform activity in human neocortex. J Clin Neurophysiol 2008;25(6):321–30.
12. Stead M, Bower M, Brinkmann BH, et al. Microseizures and the spatiotemporal scales of human partial epilepsy. Brain 2010;133(9):2789–97.
13. Ives JR, Thompson CJ, Gloor P. Seizure monitoring: a new tool in electroencephalography. Electroencephalogr Clin Neurophysiol 1976;41(4):422–7.
14. Gotman J. Automatic recognition of epileptic seizures in the EEG. Electroencephalogr Clin Neurophysiol 1982;54(5):530–40.
15. Gotman J. Automatic seizure detection: improvements and evaluation. Electroencephalogr Clin Neurophysiol 1990;76(4):317–24.
16. Qu H, Gotman J. A patient-specific algorithm for the detection of seizure onset in long-term EEG monitoring: possible use as a warning device. IEEE Trans Biomed Eng 1997;44(2):115–22.
17. Qu H, Gotman J. Improvement in seizure detection performance by automatic adaptation to the EEG of each patient. Electroencephalogr Clin Neurophysiol 1993;86(2):79–87.
18. Murro AM, King DW, Smith JR, et al. Computerized seizure detection of complex partial seizures. Electroencephalogr Clin Neurophysiol 1991;79(4):330–3.
19. Harding GW. An Automated seizure monitoring system for patients with indwelling recording electrodes. Electroencephalogr Clin Neurophysiol 1993; 86(6):428–37.
20. Osorio I, Frei MG, Wilkinson SB. Real-time automated detection and quantitative analysis of seizures and short-term prediction of clinical onset. Epilepsia 1998;39(6):615–27.
21. Osorio I, Frei MG, Giftakis J, et al. Performance reassessment of a real-time seizure-detection algorithm on long ECoG series. Epilepsia 2002;43(12):1522–35.
22. Haykin S. Neural networks: a comprehensive foundation. 2nd edition. New Jersey: Prentice Hall; 1998.
23. Pradhan N, Sadasivan PK, Arunodaya GR. Detection of seizure activity in EEG by an artificial neural network: a preliminary study. Comput Biomed Res 1996;29(4):303–13.

24. Weng W, Khorasani K. An adaptive structure neural networks with application to EEG automatic seizure detection. Neural Netw 1996;9(7):1223–40.

25. Webber WR, Lesser RP, Richardson RT, et al. An approach to seizure detection using an artificial neural network (ANN). Electroencephalogr Clin Neurophysiol 1996;98(4):250–72.

26. Gabor AJ, Leach RR, Dowla FU. Automated seizure detection using a self-organizing neural network. Electroencephalogr Clin Neurophysiol 1996;99(3):257–66.

27. Gabor AJ. Seizure detection using a self-organizing neural network: validation and comparison with other detection strategies. Electroencephalogr Clin Neurophysiol 1998;107(1):27–32.

28. Nandan M, Talathi SS, Myers S, et al. Support vector machines for seizure detection in an animal model of chronic epilepsy. J Neural Eng 2010;7(3):036001.

29. Adeli H, Zhou Z, Dadmehr N. Analysis of EEG records in an epileptic patient using wavelet transform. J Neurosci Methods 2003;123(1):69–87.

30. Sartoretto F, Ermani M. Automatic detection of epileptiform activity by single-level wavelet analysis. Clin Neurophysiol 1999;110(2):239–49.

31. Nam H, Yim TG, Han SK, et al. Independent component analysis of ictal EEG in medial temporal lobe epilepsy. Epilepsia 2002;43(2):160–4.

32. Hoeve MJ, Zwaag van der BJ, Burik van M, et al. Detecting epileptic seizure activity in the EEG by independent component analysis. In: ProRISC 14th Workshop on Circuits, Systems and Signal Processing. Veldhoven, the Netherlands, November 26–27, 2003. p. 373–82.

33. Subasi A, Gursoy MI. EEG signal classification using PCA, ICA, LDA and support vector machines. Expert Syst Appl 2010;37(12):8659–66.

34. Faul S, Boylan G, Connolly S, et al. An evaluation of automated neonatal seizure detection methods. Clin Neurophysiol 2005;116(7):1533–41.

35. Deburchgraeve W, Cherian PJ, De Vos M, et al. Automated neonatal seizure detection mimicking a human observer reading EEG. Clin Neurophysiol 2008;119(11):2447–54.

36. Comon P. Independent component analysis: a new concept? Elsevier. Signal Processing 1994;36(3):287–314.

37. Hyvarinen A, Karhunen J, Oja E. Independent component analysis. New York: John Wiley & Sons, Inc; 2001.

38. James CJ, Hesse CW. Independent component analysis for biomedical signals. Physiol Meas 2005;26:R15–39.

39. Makeig S, Westerfield M, Townsend J, et al. Functionally independent components of early event-related potentials in a visual spatial attention task. Philos Trans R Soc Lond B Biol Sci 1999;354(1387):1135–44.

40. Makeig S, Jung T, Ghahremani D, et al. Independent component analysis of simulated ERP data. In: Nakada T, editor. Integrated human brain science: theory,

method, applications. Amsterdam, Netherlands: Elsevier Science B.V; 2000. p. 1–24.

41. Makeig S, Bell AJ, Jung TP, et al. Independent component analysis of electroencephalographic data. In: Touretzky D, Mozer M, Hasselmo M, editors. Advances in neural information processing systems. Cambridge (MA): MIT Press; 1996. p. 145–51.

42. Guerrero-Mosquera C, Vazquez AN. New approach in features extraction for EEG signal detection. Conf Proc IEEE Eng Med Biol Soc 2009;2009:13–6.

43. Guerrero-Mosquera C, Trigueros AM, Franco JI, et al. New feature extraction approach for epileptic EEG signal detection using time-frequency distributions. Med Biol Eng Comput 2010;48(4):321–30.

44. Iriarte J, Urrestarazu E, Valencia M, et al. Independent component analysis as a tool to eliminate artifacts in EEG: a quantitative study. J Clin Neurophysiol 2003;20(4):249–57.

45. Jung T, Makeig S, Humphries C, et al. Removing electroencephalographic artifacts by blind source separation. Psychophysiology 2000;37(2):163–78.

46. Vigário RN. Extraction of ocular artefacts from EEG using independent component analysis. Electroencephalogr Clin Neurophysiol 1997;103(3):395–404.

47. Hyvarinen A. Fast and robust fixed-point algorithms for independent component analysis. IEEE Trans Neural Netw 1999;10(3):626–34.

48. Hyvarinen A, Oja E. Independent component analysis: algorithms and applications. Neural Netw 2000;13(4–5):411–30.

49. Bell AJ, Sejnowski TJ. An information-maximization approach to blind separation and blind deconvolution. Neural Comput 1995;7(6):1129–59.

50. Hyvarinen A, Hoyer PO, Inki M. Topographic independent component analysis. Neural Comput 2001;13(7):1527–58.

51. Jing M, Sanei S. A novel constrained topographic independent component analysis for separation of epileptic seizure signals. Comput Intell Neurosci 2007;2007:21315.

52. Jing M, Sanei S. A temporally constrained spatial ICA for separation of seizure BOLD from fMRI. In: Proc. 16th European Signal Processing Conference (EUSIPCO). Lausanne, Switzerland, August 25–29, 2008.

53. James CJ, Hesse CW. Mapping scalp topographies of rhythmic EEG activity using temporal decorrelation based constrained ICA. Conf Proc IEEE Eng Med Biol Soc 2004;2:994–7.

54. Phlypo R, Van Hese P, Hallez H, et al. Extracting the spike process from the EEG by spatially constrained ICA. Conf Proc IEEE Eng Med Biol Soc 2006;1:5286–9.

55. Cardoso JF. Multidimensional independent component analysis. In: Conf Proc ICASSP. Seattle, USA, May 12–15, 1998. p. 1941–4.

56. The Freiburg EEG database. Available at: http://epilepsy.uni-freiburg.de/freiburg-seizure-prediction-project/eeg-database. Accessed July 7, 2011.

Implanted Subdural Electrodes: Safety Issues and Complication Avoidance

Kostas N. Fountas, MD, PhD

KEYWORDS

- Complication • Edema • Electrode • Epilepsy • Hematoma
- Infection • Safety • Subdural

Epilepsy affects approximately 0.5% to 1% of the general population, and at some point approximately 20% of these patients develop medically intractable epilepsy despite adequate pharmaceutical treatment.[1] It has been estimated that 2 to 3/1000 people suffer medically refractory epilepsy, which is equivalent to 17,000 new cases per year in the United States alone.[2] More than 700,000 cases of medically refractory epilepsy exist in the United States that may be benefited from surgery.[2] Approximately 20% to 50% of these patients may have localized epilepsy and may be good candidates for resective, disconnecting, or neuromodulation procedures.[2–8] It has been shown that surgical management of these medically refractory cases significantly increases the possibility of seizure freedom, improves the postoperative quality of life, maximizes the patient's social function, and may minimize the need for anticonvulsant medications and their associated side effects.[1]

In most cases, consideration for surgical intervention requires identification and accurate localization of the epileptogenic focus or foci and any associated epileptogenic zones. Surface electroencephalography (EEG) cannot localize the epileptogenic foci in approximately 25% of the medically refractory cases.[3,5–9] In these cases in which surface EEG can identify no epileptogenic foci, or in those cases in which electrophysiologic studies

are disconcordant with imaging studies, invasive EEG is necessary for further investigation.[3,5–8,10] Invasive EEG permits more accurate and sensitive information because it is closer to the source of cortical electrical activity; it is separated only by high electrical conductivity media (cerebrospinal fluid [CSF], brain parenchyma), and thus is characterized by a high signal/noise ratio.[4–8,11–16] In addition, it can detect electrical activity from a significantly smaller cortical area than surface EEG, and has stable impedance throughout the whole recording period.[11] Furthermore, invasive EEG may provide valuable information regarding the presence of eloquent cortical areas, and thus allow accurate cortical mapping.[3,6]

The use of subdural electrodes was first described by Penfield and his coworkers in the late 1930s.[17,18] The first documented case of epidural electrode recording was performed also by Penfield, Jasper, and Hebb in 1939.[19] The use of invasive EEG monitoring started progressively increasing within the next few decades, and in the mid-1970s it became routine clinical practice for patients with medically refractory epilepsy.[10,20,21] Epidural electrodes were initially more popular, whereas strip subdural electrodes inserted via burr holes later became more frequently used.[22] The evolution of stereotactic surgery and the technological advancement of stereotactic hardware

The author has nothing to disclose.
Department of Neurosurgery, University Hospital of Larisa, School of Medicine, University of Thessaly, Biopolis, 41110 Larissa, Greece
E-mail address: fountas@med.uth.gr

neurosurgery.theclinics.com

and software allowed the wide application of depth along with subdural electrodes for invasive EEG monitoring. Likewise, the development of more biocompatible and more flexible grid electrodes led to their wide application in the preoperative investigation of patients with medically intractable epilepsy. It has been estimated that invasive recording is nowadays used in 25% to 50% of surgical epilepsy series.[23]

The wide clinical application of invasive monitoring in the preoperative evaluation of patients suffering from medically refractory epilepsy brings up the issue of safety of using invasive monitoring. It is generally accepted that subdural electrodes show higher complication rates than depth electrodes.[24] Even though subdural electrode–associated complications are rare, they can occasionally become troublesome. Thorough knowledge of all the potential complications associated with the implantation of subdural electrodes, and all subdural-related safety issues, is of paramount importance for their early recognition and prompt management.[25] Moreover, meticulous knowledge of all safety issues is mandatory for medicolegal purposes, and for appropriately informing all possible surgical candidates before obtaining their consent.[25]

This article systematically reviews the pertinent literature and identifies all safety issues associated with the implantation of subdural electrodes. All the possible complications associated with their usage are reviewed, and any predisposing factors are identified, for developing efficient strategies and protocols for avoiding complications.

MATERIAL AND METHODS

A systematic review of the English language literature was performed through the PubMed search engine. The search terms complication, depth, electrode, epidural, grid, intracranial, invasive, safety, strip, and subdural were used independently and in all possible combinations. Clinical series, miniseries, and case reports were included in our current study with no chronologic limitations. Adult, pediatric, and mixed population studies were all included in our analysis. All the recovered articles were reviewed for safety issues regarding the usage of invasive EEG monitoring, safety issues associated with the biocompatibility of the implanted electrodes, and/or the occurrence of any procedure-related or material-related complications. Special attention was paid to the study population overlap that existed in several articles, and every possible effort was made to avoid any recalculations of the reported subdural electrode–associated complications.

The type of study, the number of included patients, the type of implanted subdural electrodes, their manufacturing characteristics, the duration of invasive EEG monitoring, the perioperative management of these patients, and the observed major and/or minor complications were recorded and tabulated. Other parameters, such as the implantation surgical technique, the performing surgeon's experience, and the type of underlying epilepsy, were also examined whenever available.

The role of imaging, intracranial pressure monitoring, or other developing strategies for the avoidance or early recognition of any subdural electrode-related complications is also examined in our current study. The applied strategies of various epilepsy surgery centers for preventing any subdural electrode complications described in the examined clinical series are also critically reviewed.

RESULTS

The biocompatibility of the material of the commercially available, implantable subdural electrodes seems to raise no safety issues.[26,27] There are no reported complications, as far as we know, caused by tissue reaction either to the electrodes' contact material (platinum, silver, or stainless steel) or to the silastic material forming the matrix in which the contacts are embedded. In most of the reported cases, the contacts of the subdural electrodes are 3.97 to 5 mm in diameter, and 0.127 to 0.7 mm in thickness.[11,24,27–30] The interdiskal distance varies between 5 and 10 mm.[11,27,30] Histopathologic studies in patients undergoing invasive EEG monitoring via subdural electrodes have shown that there were no cortical changes but mild reactive leptomeningeal thickening, and mild mononuclear cell infiltration of the subarachnoid space.[26,27,31] The recently developed hybrid electrodes (**Figs. 1** and **2**), which are a combination of conventional subdural grid electrodes with microwire arrays, seem to be associated with no additional complications to the commonly occurring complications of the conventional electrodes.[32] Likewise, the use of a newer microelectrode array (Neuroport, Cyberkinetics Neurotechnology Systems Inc, Boston, MA) (**Fig. 3**), initially designed for human neuroprosthetic implantable systems, in invasive EEG recording, revealed no biocompatibility issues and no material-related brain tissue reactions.[33] This microelectrode system is a 10 by 10 array of 96 platinum electrode disks (there are no contacts at the 4 corners), embedded on a 4 mm^2 silicon base, with 400-μm interdiskal spacing.[33]

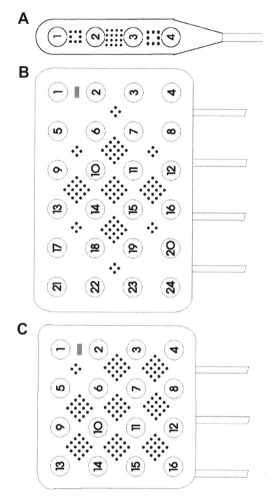

Fig. 1. A 1×4 contact strip with 32 microwires (A), a hybrid 4×6 grid with 104 microwires (B), and a hybrid 4×4 grid with 112 microwires (C). Microwires are 40-μm diameter, platinum-iridium wire spaced 1 mm apart. Clinical macrocontacts are 4 mm diameter and spaced 10 mm center to center. (*From* Van Gompel JJ, Stead SM, Giannini C, et al. Phase I trial: safety and feasibility of intracranial electroencephalography using hybrid subdural electrodes containing macro- and microelectrode arrays. Neurosurg Focus 2008; 25:2; with permission.)

Histopathologic examination of the resected cortex in these cases revealed minimal tissue reaction with mild regional microglial activation and limited scattered microhemorrhages.[33]

The development of postimplantation edema constitutes another troublesome complication of invasive EEG monitoring via subdural electrodes (**Table 1**).[14,23,25,29,30,34–39] Its occurrence varies among previously reported series between 0.5% and 14%.[14,29,34–37] Fountas and Smith[25] reported a fatal case caused by the development of uncontrollable edema and intracranial hypertension

in a patient with subdural grid implantation, whereas the overall incidence of postimplantation-increased intracranial pressure (ICP) was 1.1% in their series. Likewise, Wong and colleagues[30] reported a 2.8% death rate in their series, caused by the development of postimplantation edema and subsequent cerebral infarction. Burneo and colleagues[23] reported that transient neurologic deficits secondary to focal brain edema occurred in 1.3% of their cases. Lee and colleagues[38] reported that 4.9% of their cases developed acute cerebral infarction caused by edema formation. Giussani and colleagues[39] reported brain edema development in 8% of their patients. Van Gompel and colleagues[32] reported that 4.1% of their patients undergoing hybrid subdural electrode implantation showed acute neurologic deterioration caused by severe cerebral edema development.

The development of postoperative epidural hematoma (EDH) was one of the most common and acute complications in the previously published series, with an incidence varying between 1.8% and 2.5%.[25,34,35,39–41] Immediate surgical evacuation was necessary in most large hematomas accompanied by an acute change in the patient's neurologic condition.[25] However, there are several reports that identify the formation of rim EDH after subdural grid implantation, which required no surgical evacuation.[42–45]

Similarly, the development of postimplantation subdural hematoma (SDH) has been reported in 1.1% to 14%.[23–25,29,30,32,35–37,39,46] Fountas and Smith[25] reported a 1.1% incidence of SDH in their series. However, surgical evacuation was necessary in only 0.5% of their cases.[25] Van Gompel and colleagues[32] reported a 4.1% incidence of small-size SDHs requiring no surgical intervention in their series with hybrid subdural electrodes. Likewise, Wong and colleagues[30] reported SDH formation in 5.6% of their cases, whereas Burneo and colleagues[23] reported a slightly higher incidence of SDH: 13% in patients with grids and 3% in patients with strips. Giussani and colleagues[39] found in their series that 65% of their pediatric patients had an average midline shift of 4 mm on their postoperative computed tomography (CT) scans. However, only 5% of their cases required surgical evacuation of their hematomas.[39] Bozkurt and colleagues[47] reported a case of circumscribed subelectrode hematoma with no subdural component, which was not visible on the obtained CT scan but became evident during electrode removal. They assumed that tearing of a cortical vein was responsible for their unusual finding.[47]

The implantation of subdural electrodes and the prolonged invasive EEG monitoring have

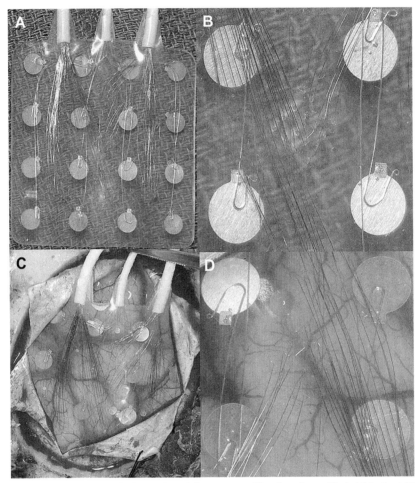

Fig. 2. The hybrid grid for intracranial monitoring. (*A*) Low-magnification view of hybrid 4×4 grid before implantation. (*B*) High-magnification view of the grid subunit. Note how 4 macroelectrodes surround a diamond-shaped and centered 4×4 grid of microwires. (*C*) Low-magnification view of implanted grid in a patient. (*D*) High-magnification view of grid subunit over human cortex. Note the improved spatial resolution of microwires compared with macroelectrodes. (*From* Van Gompel JJ, Stead SM, Giannini C, et al. Phase I trial: safety and feasibility of intracranial electroencephalography using hybrid subdural electrodes containing macro-and microelectrode arrays. Neurosurg Focus 2008;25:3; with permission.)

been associated with infection development.[12,14,23–25,29,30,34,35,37,39,40,48–52] The reported infection rates range between 1.1% and 17%.[12,14,23–25,29,30,34,35,37,39,40,48–52] Fountas and Smith[25] reported a low infection rate of 1.1% in their series. Similarly, Burneo and colleagues[23] found that an infection was encountered in 1.3% of their cases. Wong and colleagues[30] reported a slightly higher infection rate of 2.8% in their cohort. Several clinical series have been reported with infection rates ranging from 0% to 2.8%.[23,27,36,41,46,51,52] Characteristically, Van Gompel and colleagues[32] and Waziri and colleagues,[33] in their series of patients with hybrid and microelectrodes respectively, found that none of their patients developed any infections. However, many clinical investigators

have reported significantly higher infection rates, ranging between 3.3% and 17% of their patients.[34,35,40,48–50,53,54] Lee and colleagues[35] reported an infection rate of 4.1%, whereas Musleh and colleagues[12] found an infection rate of 6.9% in their pediatric series. Hamer and colleagues[34] reported one of the highest infection rates, of 12.1%, in their retrospective study.

The occurrence of postimplantation CSF leakage constitutes a common condition in patients undergoing invasive EEG monitoring, and may increase the risk of postoperative hematoma and infection.[25] In addition, it has been associated with difficulties in EEG monitoring and recording.[27] Fountas and Smith[25] reported no incidence of postoperative CSF leakage through the electrode

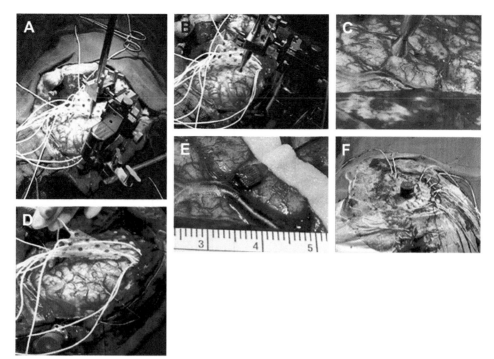

Fig. 3. Representative intraoperative photographs showing elements of the microarray insertion procedure. (*A*) Setup of the surgical field after craniotomy, dural opening, and preliminary grid insertion. The positioning device for the impactor wand has been attached to a Greenberg retractor system. (*B*) Close-up view of the positioning device, showing multidimensional capability for fine-tuning of the impactor wand. (*C*) Close-up view of the impactor wand near the cortical target, in preparation for microarray implantation. (*D*) View of microarray after transpial insertion and stabilization with silk sutures to the dural edge. The device pedestal has been fixed to the cranium at the edge of the craniotomy. (*E*) Close-up view of the implanted microarray, showing mild subpial hemorrhage. (*F*) Final appearance of the device pedestal after wound closure. In this patient, the pedestal was brought through the scalp flap via a separate stab incision. (*From* Waziri A, Schevon CA, Cappell J, et al. Initial surgical experience with a dense cortical microarray in epileptic patients undergoing craniotomy for subdural electrode implantation. Neurosurgery 2009;64:542; with permission.)

cable exiting sites in their series. In contrast, Adelson and colleagues[46] reported an 8.6% incidence of persistent CSF leakage in their series. Swartz and colleagues[27] reported persistent CSF leakage in 19% of their cases, whereas Onal and colleagues[36] reported CSF leakage in 20% of their patients. Waziri and colleagues[33] reported that CSF leakage was frequent in their series of microelectrode implantation.

The occurrence of other than the habitual type of seizures after a subdural grid electrode implantation has been previously reported.[25,55,56] Fountas and Smith[25] reported that the incidence of nonhabitual seizure recording was 2.7% in their series. Similarly, Malow and colleagues[56] reported a case of nonhabitual seizures in a patient with an SDH caused by a subdural grid implantation. Although the recording of atypical seizures cannot be considered a complication of invasive monitoring, it can be misleading and, if not adequately identified, it may have a significant impact on the patient's surgical treatment and the overall outcome.

Minor complications such as headache, nausea, transient increase of the patient's temperature, persistent fever, aseptic meningitis, neck stiffness, increased prothrombin time, hyponatremia, delirious state development, leucocytosis, mild sleepiness during the first postoperative days, migraine headache, and typical postoperative headache are associated with the implantation of subdural electrodes.[12,23,25,27,32,34,57,58] However, detailed information regarding the exact incidence of such minor complications is limited, because, for a long period of time, most of these complications were considered to be expected conditions.[25,34] Van Gompel and colleagues[32] reported that 8.3% of their patients developed low-grade fever, 4.1% developed hyponatremia, and 45.8% developed leucocytosis after undergoing implantation of hybrid subdural electrodes. Burneo and colleagues[23] reported that 1.3% of their patients developed symptoms of aseptic meningitis. Similarly, Musleh and colleagues[12] found that 3.4% of their patients developed low-grade fever, and another 3.4%

Table 1
Demographic data and incidence rates of the most commonly occurring subdural electrode–associated complications

Series	Patient Population	No. of Patients	Implanted Electrodes	Type of Electrodes	No. of Days Monitored (Mean Duration)	EDH Rate (%)	SDH Rate (%)	Infection Rate (%)	Edema Incidence (%)
Wyler et al,[50] 1984	Adult	28	30	Strips	<21	None	None	3.6	None
Rosenbaum et al,[4] 1986	Adult	50	N/A	Strips	2–21 (7)	None	None	None	None
Wyllie et al,[49] 1988	Pediatric adult	23 38	N/A	Grids and strips	9–32 (17) 7–32 (17)	None	None	17 13	Few cases (no exact number)
Spencer et al,[14] 1990	Adult	47	104	Grids and strips	<14	None	None	1.5	1.5
Wyler et al,[52] 1991	Adult	350	350	Strips	2–28 (4.5)	None	None	0.8	None
Behrens et al,[51] 1994	Pediatric and adult	158	N/A	Grids and strips	N/A	None	0.6	2.5	None
Adelson et al,[46] 1995	Pediatric	31	46	Grids and strips	3–23 (11)	None	2.1	None	None
Swartz et al,[27] 1996	Adult	55	58	Grids and strips	3–16 (10)	None	None	None	None
Silberbusch et al,[37] 1998	Pediatric and adult	51	N/A	Grids	N/A	None	7.8	1.9	None
Wiggins et al,[40] 1999	Adult	38	53	Grids and strips	9–28 (13.4)	1.8	None	5.6	None
Zaccariotti et al,[41] 1999	Pediatric	44	45	Grids	2–18 (8.4)	2.2	None	None	None
Lee et al,[35] 2000	Pediatric and adult	49	50	Grids	5–24 (12)	2	8	4	2
Rudesker and	Pediatric and adult	205	121 strips	Grids and strips	N/A	0.5	2.9	1.9	None

Study									
Onal et al,[36] 2003	Pediatric	35	N/A	Grids and strips	N/A	None	14	None	14
Bauman et al,[48] 2005	Pediatric	15	N/A	Grids and strips	4–8 (6.5)	None	None	6.7	None
Musleh et al,[12] 2006	Pediatric	29	3700 subdural contacts	Grids and strips	(97.1 ± 0.5)	None	None	6.9	None
Burneo et al,[23] 2006	Adult	116	Mean: 8 strips per case	Grids and strips	3–29 (12.3)	None	None	1.3	None
Fountas and Smith,[25] 2007	Adult	185	318 grids 226 strips	Grids and strips	2–25 (10.8)	1.6	1.1	1.1	1.1
Van Gompel et al,[32] 2008	Adult	24	Mean:56.7 ± 27.4 Range:16–96	Hybrid	(7 ± 3) 3–15	None	4.1	None	None
Van Gompel et al,[29] 2008	Pediatric and adult	189	198 grids	Grids	(8 ± 04)	None	3	2.5	13.8
Lee et al,[38] 2008	Pediatric and adult	41	51grids	Grids and strips	(5) 1–7	None	2.4	None	4.8
Waziri et al,[33] 2009	Adult	7	7	Microelectrodes	(10.1) 3–28	None	None	None	None
Wong et al,[30] 2009	Adult	71	Median: 62 Range:8–164	Grids and strips	(11) 7–14	None	5.6	2.8	1.4
Placantonakis et al,[28] 2010	Adult	26	N/A	Strips	(8.2)	None	None	None	None

Abbreviations: EDH, epidural hematoma; SDH, subdural hematoma.

had increased prothrombin time. Swartz and colleagues[27] reported that the incidence of typical postoperative headache was 15%, the incidence of migraine headache after implantation was 5.2%, and the incidence of nausea was 4%. Furthermore, 41% of their patients presented low-grade fever and another 5.2% high-grade fever.[27] Hamer and colleagues[34] reported that 0.5% of their patients became delirious after a subdural electrode implantation.

Various systemic complications, not directly associated with the subdural electrode implantation, are found in the literature.[25,40,41] Zaccariotti and colleagues[41] have reported the incidence of such complications to be 2.2% in their series, whereas Wiggins and colleagues[40] reported 5.6% incidence in their cohort. Most of them are respiratory system complications.[40,41] Likewise, Fountas and Smith[25] reported a case with fatal outcome, caused by the development of stiff lung syndrome after subdural grid implantation.

DISCUSSION

The included studies show great heterogeneity in their populations, their methodology, the type and the manufacturers of the used subdural electrodes, and the surgical implantation techniques.[12,13,21,23,24,27–30,32–35,37–39,41,49,50,57,59] The experience of the epilepsy surgeon constitutes another confounding factor, because this was a highly variable parameter between the reviewed studies and, in a few long-term studies, existed even within the same study.[10,34] Furthermore, the perioperative management of patients undergoing long-term invasive EEG monitoring varied significantly, not only between different clinical series but occasionally in the same study in different study periods. In addition, the monitoring period as well as the number and the configuration of the implanted electrodes significantly varied between the reviewed clinical series. Therefore, comparative analysis of their results and the extraction of any statistically powerful conclusions of such a comparison are impossible.

The biocompatibility of the implanted subdural electrodes and the potential brain parenchyma reaction to the implanted foreign body has been an important issue.[26] Several experimental animal studies have shown that direct electrical cortical stimulation may cause damage to the underlying cortex and regional disruption of the blood-brain barrier.[26] However, human histopathologic studies have shown that chronic implantation of subdural electrodes and cortical stimulation of the underlying human cortex caused only a mild diffuse reactive gliosis.[26,27] This was accompanied by

a mild increase of mononuclear inflammatory cells in the subarachnoid space, as well as an increase in the concentration of periodic acid-Schiff–positive granules in cortical layers I and II.[26] It has been postulated that these minor changes were the result of a tissue reaction to the silastic matrix of the implanted subdural electrodes.[26] The necessity for recording electrical activity from smaller cortical areas, and also recording micro-seizures and microepileptiform activity, led to the recent development of microelectrodes and hybrid electrodes.[32,33] These implantable subdural and/or subpial electrodes can record electrical activity almost from cortical macrocolumns, as well as hippocampal fast ripples.[32,33] The histopathologic studies performed so far have confirmed that there are only mild and spatially limited tissue reactions (microglial reaction, microhemorrhage formation).[33]

The development of postimplantation edema may occasionally be a serious complication. The exact pathophysiologic mechanism for subdural electrode–associated edema remains unclear. It has been postulated that compression of large cortical veins or adjacent venous sinuses caused by large subdural grids may be responsible for the development of edema.[36] The net mechanical effect of a large or multiple implanted subdural grids may increase the volume of the intracranial components, and thus may crucially increase the ICP. This theory seems to be the underlying pathophysiologic mechanism, especially in children. Various surgical strategies have been proposed for preventing the development of postimplantation edema. Onal and colleagues[36] suggested that careful implantation of the subdural electrodes by avoiding compression of cortical veins, performance of an extensive duroplasty, and hinging craniotomy may minimize the risk of intracranial hypertension. Similarly, Bauman and colleagues[48] suggested the performance of a temporary decompressive craniectomy for avoiding postimplantation intracranial hypertension. However, Van Gompel and colleagues[29] found that decompressive craniectomy did not prevent the development of postimplantation edema. The role of systematic administration of steroids remains to be proved. Several centers routinely administer steroids for 72 hours, at least after the implantation, and then progressively taper them off.[23,25,27,29,30,34] The benefit of the steroid administration should be weighed against their potential side effects and the increased risk of infection, particularly in patients with prolonged invasive EEG monitoring. In the past, the systematic administration of mannitol was proposed as a measure for minimizing the risk of postimplantation edema.[25] However, Etame and colleagues[60] found that mannitol paradoxically increases the grid-associated mass effect. Numerous series have identified the increased number of implanted grids, their large size, the coverage of previously damaged cortical areas, and the patients' young age as predisposing factors for developing edema.[24,25,30,38,61] In this particular group of implanted patients, it may be beneficial to consider administration of steroids, performing duroplasty and/or craniectomy, and inserting an ICP monitor for early detection and prompt management of the development of edema.

The incidence of postimplantation hematomas seems to be higher than previously reported in patients with subdural electrodes.[39,62] The routine administration of postoperative CT scan has indicated that the occurrence of mostly SDH or subdural fluid collection is higher than that reported in older series, because most of these subdural collections remain clinically silent and can easily remain undetected.[39,62] Giussani and colleagues[39] found that the use of an early postoperative CT scan may recognize small SDHs but cannot predict the development of symptomatic hemorrhagic complications. The exact pathophysiologic mechanism responsible for the development of epidural or subdural postimplantation hematomas in the absence of any intraoperative bleeding has remained unclear.[25] The displacement of the implanted grid over the underlying cortex during seizures, especially violent seizures, can theoretically injure the adjacent cortical bridging veins and cause the formation of an SDH.[25,35] Moreover, asymmetric electrode implantation may be responsible for the development of an SDH because of acute alteration of the ICP dynamics.[35] Similarly, CSF leakage around the electrode exit sites can produce a pressure shift toward the side of the implanted subdural electrode, with subsequent brain shift and tearing of a bridging vein, leading to an SDH.[35] The occurrence of SDHs seems to be higher among adult patients.[34] This may be explained by the increased parenchyma plasticity and the decreased vascular structure rigidity of the pediatric brain.[34] The insertion of a subdural drain could theoretically minimize the incidence of postoperative SDH.[30,35] Lee and colleagues[35] reported that, after using a subdural drain on a routine basis, they noticed no cases of SDH in their patients. However, the insertion of a subdural drain can be responsible for ICP changes, and further brain shift by draining CSF, and thus may increase the chance of SDH formation. The development of a new generation of subdural electrodes with more rounded corners, which will be embedded in material that is more flexible and easy to contour, may further minimize the occurrence of vascular mechanical trauma, and subsequently the development of postoperative hematomas.

The development of postimplantation infection is a well-described complication of invasive EEG monitoring, which occasionally may have severe neurologic consequences, and may frequently alter the original plan for resective surgery. Wiggins and colleagues,[40] in their prospective study, found that the associated risk of infection increases significantly when more than 100 electrode contacts are implanted, when more than 10 exiting electrode cables are present, and/or when the electrodes remain implanted for more than 14 days. Likewise, Hamer and colleagues[34] concluded that an increased number of electrodes (>60 contacts), prolonged monitoring time (>10 days), and the presence of burr holes additional to the performed craniotomy increased the risk of infection. However, Wyllie and colleagues,[49] in their large clinical series, found that duration of monitoring had no impact on the observed infection rate. Similarly, Musleh and colleagues[12] concluded from their pediatric series that the number of implanted electrodes, the number of exiting cables, and the duration of monitoring played no role in their infection rate. However, they found that their infection rate was increased in cases of reimplantation.[12] Numerous clinical series agree that the surgical implantation technique significantly influences the observed infection rate.[10,34,49] Wyllie and colleagues[49] found that the infection rate was not significantly different between pediatric and adult patients in their series.

The observed subdural electrode–associated infections may result in meningitis and/or cerebritis, osteomyelitis, skin abscess, or systemic sepsis.[25,30,34,49] Various pathogens have been implicated in the development of postimplantation infections.[30,34,49] However, Staphylococcus and Streptococcus species are usually responsible for most of the observed infections.[30,34,49] The systematic administration and the duration of antibiotic coverage in patients undergoing subdural grid/strip electrode implantation constitute another controversial point in the management of these patients. Administration of antibiotics throughout the invasive EEG monitoring period is followed in several epilepsy centers.[25,27,30,34,40,41,46,48] However, Wyler and colleagues[52] found in their prospective study that the administration of antibiotics throughout the invasive monitoring period had no impact on the observed infection rate. Their infection rate among patients without antibiotic coverage was not significantly different from that observed in patients covered with antibiotics.[52] However, only strip electrodes through burr holes were implanted in their series, and no craniotomies were performed for electrode implantation.[52] Further improvement of the biomedical properties of the implanted electrodes (slow-releasing antibiotic electrode, pathogen adherence–resistant electrode), along with lege artis surgical implantation technique, including watertight externalization of the electrode cables with skin tunneling remotely from the craniotomy skin incision, may further minimize the risk infection in the future.

Although persistent CSF leakage may not be considered a complication per se, it may increase the risk of developing other potential serious complications, such as postoperative hematoma, worsening of the implanted electrodes' mass effect, postoperative infection, brain edema worsening, and EEG recording dysfunction. Several measures have been periodically proposed for avoiding or minimizing the chance of postimplantation CSF leakage. Skin tunneling of the exiting electrode tails, the application of collodion at the exiting site, and the achievement of a watertight skin closure by applying a figure-of-eight stitch at the exiting site, are a few of the strategies reported in the pertinent literature.[12,27] Weinand and Oommen,[63] in their prospective clinical study, showed that the insertion of a lumbar drain, and continuous postoperative CSF drainage could decrease the incidence of CSF leakage through the electrode cable exiting sites, and thus may minimize the risk of infection or other complications. Further designing improvement of the newer generation subdural and/or subpial microelectrodes may decrease the incidence of postoperative CSF leakage.

The occurrence and the recording of nonhabitual seizures in a few rare occasions have been associated with the formation of a thin layer of blood underneath the implanted subdural grid.[25,55] This subelectrode rim blood clot was not visible on the obtained CT scans, but was intraoperatively identified.[25,55] No macroscopic or microscopic changes were found in the resected cortex, lying underneath the implanted subdural grid and generating the nonhabitual seizure activity.[25,55] Knowledge of the possibility of recording nonhabitual seizures is essential for the accurate interpretation of the recorded invasive EEG, and the prompt decision-making process for surgical resection.

Although the occurrence of minor complications is well established with the implantation of subdural electrodes, its actual incidence cannot be calculated. It is also generally accepted that these minor complications become problematic in an extremely limited number of cases. However, such morbidities may occasionally have

legal ramifications.[58] In addition, uncomfortable patients are less cooperative, usually require more intensive nursing care, and are generally more restless, resulting in degradation of the quality of the obtained EEG recording.[58] Sahjpaul and colleagues,[58] in a prospective, randomized, controlled study examining the role of dexamethasone administration in decreasing the incidence of minor complications, found that perioperative administration of dexamethasone significantly decreased the incidence of postoperative nausea, and significantly lowered the patient's postimplantation low-grade fever. They also documented that postoperative pain (measured by using the Visual Analog Scale), amount of required pain medication, and meningismus were less common among patients receiving systematic dexamethasone, compared with those without dexamethasone.[58] However, this difference did not reach the levels of statistical significance in their study.[58] They concluded that the beneficial effects of dexamethasone seem to be delayed in onset, and of limited duration, and that further clinical studies are required for determining the ideal steroid dosage.[58]

The patients undergoing subdural electrode implantation may develop systemic complications secondary to their surgical procedure and their postoperative immobilization, which are not directly associated with the implanted electrodes.[25,40,41] Most implanted patients experience multiple seizures, frequently violent, which may occasionally evolve to status epilepticus. Therefore, the associated general morbidity during the invasive EEG monitoring period may be high. Measures for maintaining a good respiratory condition, minimizing the chance of deep vein thrombosis, and keeping under control any other comorbidity parameters are of paramount importance for avoiding or minimizing such systemic complications. Further improvement in the design of the newer microelectrodes by extending the length of the pedestal cable, and by decreasing the size of the pedestal egress site, may help by making easier the postimplantation mobilization of these patients. Moreover, the development of more sensitive subdural and/or subpial electrodes may increase their recording sensitivity and accuracy, and thus may help in decreasing the length of the monitoring period, and may minimize the risk of any general systemic complications.

SUMMARY

The use of invasive EEG monitoring via subdural electrodes constitutes a highly sensitive methodology for the preoperative investigation of patients suffering medically refractory epilepsy. The implantation of conventional subdural strip and/or grid electrodes provides the opportunity for close examination of the cortical electrical activity, better signal/noise ratio compared with the noninvasive EEG, and small cortical area coverage. However, subdural electrode implantation has been associated with the occurrence of rare, but occasionally troublesome, complications. Thorough knowledge of all subdural electrode safety issues, and meticulous understanding of the incidence of all potential complications and their underlying pathophysiologic mechanisms, may help in developing strategies for avoiding or minimizing their occurrence, and thus may improve the patients' overall outcomes.

Conventional subdural grid and/or strip electrodes show no biocompatibility issues. The development of postimplantation edema, postoperative subdural or epidural hematomas, postoperative infections, persistent CSF leakage, and recording of nonhabitual seizures along with headache, signs of meningismus, and/or low-grade fever are the most commonly encountered complications in patients undergoing subdural electrode implantation and invasive EEG monitoring.

Novel subdural and subpial hybrid and microelectrodes have been developed for recording local field potentials, microseizures, and microepileptiform activity. These electrodes may record from smaller cortical areas, providing a more sensitive tool for the preoperative evaluation of patients with medically refractory epilepsy. The early reported experience from their clinical application seems to suggest complication rates similar to those of conventional subdural electrodes. Further clinical evaluation of these next-generation electrodes is necessary for accurately evaluating their safety and their clinical efficacy.

REFERENCES

1. Wiebe S, Blume WT, Girvin JP, et al. A randomized, controlled trial of surgery for temporal-lobe epilepsy. N Engl J Med 2001;345:311–8.
2. Spire WJ, Jobst BC, Thadani VM, et al. Robotic image-guided depth electrode implantation in the evaluation of medically intractable epilepsy. Neurosurg Focus 2008;25:E19.
3. Gloor P. Contributions of electroencephalography and electrocorticography to the neurosurgical treatment of epilepsies. Adv Neurol 1975;8:59–106.
4. Rosenbaum TJ, Laxer KD, Vessely M, et al. Subdural electrodes for seizure focus localization. Neurosurgery 1986;19:73–81.
5. Wyler AR. The role of depth and subdural electrodes in the workup of surgical candidates. In: Miller JW, Silbergeld DL, editors. Epilepsy surgery: principles and controversies. New York: Taylor & Francis; 2006. p. 280–2.
6. Benbadis SR, Wyllie E, Bingaman WE. Intracranial electroencephalography and localization studies. In: Wyllie E, editor. The treatment of epilepsy: principles and practice. 4th edition. Philadelphia: Lippincott Williams & Wilkins; 2006. p. 1059–67.
7. Ebner A, Luders HO. Subdural electrodes. In: Luders HO, Comair YG, editors. Epilepsy surgery. 2nd edition. Philadelphia: Lippincott Williams & Wilkins; 2001. p. 593–6.
8. Arroyo S, Lesser RP, Awad IA, et al. Subdural and epidural grids and strips. In: Engel J Jr, editor. Surgical treatment of the epilepsies. 2nd edition. Philadelphia: Lippincott-Raven; 1996. p. 377–86.
9. Spencer SS, Guimaraes P, Shewmon A. Intracranial electrodes. In: Engel J Jr, Pedley TA, editors. Epilepsy: a comprehensive textbook. New York: Lippincott-Raven; 1998. p. 1719–48.
10. Nair DR, Burgess R, McIntyre CC, et al. Chronic subdural electrodes in the management of epilepsy. Clin Neurophysiol 2008;119:11–28.
11. Cooper R, Winter AI, Crow HJ, et al. Comparison of subcortical, cortical and scalp activity using chronically indwelling electrodes in man. Electroencephalogr Clin Neurophysiol 1965;18:217–28.
12. Musleh W, Yassari R, Hecox K, et al. Low incidence of subdural grid-related complications in prolonged pediatric EEG monitoring. Pediatr Neurosurg 2006; 42:284–7.
13. Dubeau F, McLachlan RS. Invasive electro-graphic recording techniques in temporal lobe epilepsy. Can J Neurol Sci 2000;27(Suppl 1):S29–34.
14. Spencer SS, Spencer DD, Williamson PD, et al. Combined depth and subdural electrode investigation in uncontrolled epilepsy. Neurology 1990;40: 74–9.
15. van Veelen CW, Debets RM, van Huffelen AC, et al. Combined use of subdural and intracerebral electrodes in preoperative evaluation of epilepsy. Neurosurgery 1990;26:93–101.
16. Luders H, Awad I, Burgess R, et al. Subdural electrodes in the presurgical evaluation for surgery of epilepsy. Epilepsy Res Suppl 1992;5:147–56.
17. Morris HH III, Lüders H. Electrodes. Electroencephalogr Clin Neurophysiol Suppl 1985;37:3–26.
18. Penfield W, Jasper H. Epilepsy and the functional anatomy of the human brain. Boston: Little, Brown; 1954.
19. Almeida AN, Martinez V, Feindel W. The first case of invasive EEG monitoring for the surgical treatment of epilepsy: historical significance and context. Epilepsia 2005;46:1082–5.
20. van Veelen CW, Debets RM. Functional neurosurgery in the treatment of epilepsy in the Netherlands. Acta Neurochir 1993;124:7–10.

21. Jayaker P, Duchowny M, Resnick T. Subdural monitoring in the evaluation of children for epilepsy surgery. J Child Neurol 1994;9:2S61–6.

22. Ludwig BI, Van Buren J. Depth and direct cortical recording in seizure disorders of extratemporal origin. Neurology 1976;26:1085–99.

23. Burneo JG, Steven DA, McLachan RS, et al. Morbidity association with the use of intracranial electrodes for epilepsy surgery. Can J Neurol Sci 2006;33:223–7.

24. Rydenhag B, Silander HC. Complications of epilepsy surgery after 654 procedures in Sweden, September 1990–1995: a multicenter study based on the Swedish National Epilepsy Surgery Register. Neurosurgery 2001;49:51–6.

25. Fountas KN, Smith JR. Subdural electrode-associated complications: a 20-year experience. Stereotact Funct Neurosurg 2007;85:264–72.

26. Gordon B, Lesser RP, Rance NE, et al. Parameters for direct cortical electrical stimulation in the human: histopathologic confirmation. Electroencephalogr Clin Neurophysiol 1990;75:371–7.

27. Swartz BE, Rich JR, Dwan PS, et al. The safety and efficacy of chronically implanted subdural electrodes: a prospective study. Surg Neurol 1996;46:87–93.

28. Placantonakis DG, Shariff S, Lafaille F, et al. Bilateral intracranial electrodes for lateralizing intractable epilepsy: efficacy, risk, and outcome. Neurosurgery 2010;66:274–83.

29. Van Gompel JJ, Worrell GA, Bell ML, et al. Intracranial electroencephalography with subdural grid electrodes: techniques, complications, and outcomes. Neurosurgery 2008;63:498–505.

30. Wong CH, Birkett J, Byth K, et al. Risk factors for complications during intracranial electrode recording in presurgical evaluation of drug resistant partial epilepsy. Acta Neurochir (Wien) 2009;151(1):37–50.

31. Stephan CL, Kepes JJ, SantaCruz K, et al. Spectrum of clinical and histopathologic response to intracranial electrodes: from multifocal aseptic meningitis to multifocal hypersensitivity-type meningovasculitis. Epilepsia 2001;42:895–901.

32. Van Gompel JJ, Mathew Stead S, Giannini C, et al. Phase I trial: safety and feasibility of intracranial electroencephalography using hybrid subdural electrodes containing macro-and microelectrode arrays. Neurosurg Focus 2008;25:E23.

33. Waziri A, Schevon CA, Cappell J, et al. Initial surgical experience with a dense cortical microarray in epileptic patients undergoing craniotomy for subdural electrode implantation. Neurosurgery 2009;64:540–5.

34. Hamer HM, Morris HH, Mascha EJ, et al. Complications of invasive video-EEG monitoring with subdural grid electrodes. Neurology 2002;58:97–103.

35. Lee WS, Lee JK, Lee SA, et al. Complications and results of subdural grid electrode implantation in epilepsy surgery. Surg Neurol 2000;54:346–51.

36. Onal C, Otsubo H, Araki T, et al. Complications of invasive subdural grid monitoring in children with epilepsy. J Neurosurg 2003;98:1017–26.

37. Silberbusch MA, Rothman MI, Bergey GK, et al. Subdural grid implantation for intracranial EEG recording: CT and MR appearance. AJNR Am J Neuroradiol 1998;19:1089–93.

38. Lee JH, Hwang YS, Shin JJ, et al. Surgical complications of epilepsy surgery procedures: experience of 179 procedures in a single institute. J Korean Neurosurg Soc 2008;44:234–9.

39. Giussani C, Filardi T, Bunyaratavej K, et al. Is postoperative CT scanning predictive of subdural electrode placement complications in pediatric epileptic patients? Pediatr Neurosurg 2009;45:345–9.

40. Wiggins GC, Elisevich K, Smith BJ. Morbidity and infection in combined subdural grid and strip electrode investigation for intractable epilepsy. Epilepsy Res 1999;37:73–80.

41. Zaccariotti VA, Pannek HW, Holthausen H, et al. Evaluation with subdural plates in children. Neurol Res 1999;21:463–74.

42. Kelly DF, Nikas DL, Becker DP. Diagnosis and treatment of moderate and severe head injuries in adults. In: Youmans JR, editor. Neurological surgery, 4th edition. vol. 3. Philadelphia: WB Saunders; 1996. p. 1618–707.

43. Aldrich EF, Eisenberg HM. Acute subdural hematoma. In: Apuzzo ML, editor. Brain surgery complication avoidance and management. New York: Churchill Livingstone; 1993. p. 1283–98.

44. Cooper PR. Post-traumatic intracranial mass lesions. In: Cooper PR, editor. Head injury. 3rd edition. Baltimore (MD): Williams & Wilkins; 1993. p. 275–329.

45. Miller JD. Evaluation and treatment of head injury in adults. Neurosurg Q 1992;2:28–43.

46. Adelson PD, Black PM, Madsen JR, et al. Use of subdural grids and strip electrodes to identify a seizure focus in children. Pediatr Neurosurg 1995;22:174–80.

47. Bozkurt G, Ayhan S, Dericioglu N, et al. An unusual complication of invasive video-EEG monitoring: subelectrode hematoma without subdural component: case report. Childs Nerv Syst 2010;26:1109–12.

48. Bauman JA, Feoli E, Romanelli P, et al. Multistage epilepsy surgery: safety, efficacy, and utility of a novel approach in pediatric extratemporal epilepsy. Neurosurgery 2005;56:318–34.

49. Wyllie E, Luders H, Morris HH III, et al. Subdural electrodes in the evaluation for epilepsy surgery in children and adults. Neuropediatrics 1988;19:80–6.

50. Wyler AR, Ojemann GA, Lettich E, et al. Subdural strip electrodes for localizing epileptogenic foci. J Neurosurg 1984;60:1195–200.

51. Behrens E, Zentner J, vanRoost D, et al. Subdural and depth electrodes in the presurgical evaluation of epilepsy. Acta Neurochir 1994;128:84–7.

52. Wyler AR, Walker G, Somes G. The morbidity of long-term seizure monitoring using subdural strip electrodes. J Neurosurg 1991;74:734–7.

53. Bruce DA, Bizzi JWJ. Surgical technique for the insertion of grids and strips for invasive monitoring in children with intractable epilepsy. Childs Nerv Syst 2000;16:724–30.

54. Uematsu S, Lesser R, Fisher R, et al. Resection of the epileptogenic area in critical cortex with the aid of a subdural electrode grid. Stereotact Funct Neurosurg 1990;54–55:34–45.

55. Fountas KN, King DW, Jenkins PD, et al. Nonhabitual seizures in patients with implanted subdural electrodes. Stereotact Funct Neurosurg 2004;82:165–8.

56. Malow BA, Sato S, Kufta CV, et al. Hematoma-related seizures detected during subdural electrode monitoring. Epilepsia 1995;36:733–5.

57. Pilcher WH, Rusyniak WG. Complications of epilepsy surgery. Neurosurg Clin N Am 1993;4:311–25.

58. Sahjpaul RL, Mahon J, Wiebe S. Dexamethasone for morbidity after subdural electrode insertion - a randomized controlled trial. Can J Neurol Sci 2003;30:340–8.

59. Siegel AM, Roberts DW, Thadani VM, et al. The role of intracranial electrode reevaluation in epilepsy patients after failed initial invasive monitoring. Epilepsia 2000;41:571–80.

60. Etame AB, Fox WC, Sagher O. Osmotic diuresis paradoxically worsens brain shift after subdural grid placement. Acta Neurochir (Wien) 2011;153:633–7.

61. Jobst BC, Williamson PD, Coughlin CT, et al. An unusual complication of intracranial electrodes. Epilepsia 2000;41(7):898–902.

62. Mocco J, Komotar RJ, Ladouceur AK, et al. Radiographic characteristics fail to predict clinical course after subdural electrode placement. Neurosurgery 2006;58:120–5.

63. Weinand ME, Oommen KJ. Lumbar cerebral spinal fluid drainage during long-term electrocorticographic monitoring with subdural strip electrodes: elimination of cerebral spinal fluid leak. Seizure 1993;2:133–6.

Focal Cooling Devices for the Surgical Treatment of Epilepsy

Matthew D. Smyth, MD[a],*, Steven M. Rothman, MD[b]

KEYWORDS

- Epilepsy • Focal cooling • Devices • Peltier • Heat sink

THE CLINICAL PROBLEM OF EPILEPSY

Humans have been affected by epilepsy for thousands of years. By the end of the twentieth century, there were several remarkable advances toward understanding and treating many of the epilepsies. Scientific speculation that some genetic epilepsies were caused by mutations in ion and voltage-gated channels was validated by a series of landmark genetic discoveries. New anticonvulsants, several with highly favorable therapeutic indices, were introduced. Sensitive magnetic resonance– and positron emission–based imaging tests emerged and rapidly evolved, revealing the focal cause of many complicated epilepsies. The once radical therapeutic option of surgical resection entered the epilepsy treatment mainstream. Yet, despite these advances, many patients are still affected by epilepsy as investigators search for more effective treatments.

Particularly problematic are the focal extratemporal epilepsies, occurring in up to half of the patients with poorly controlled seizures. Focal and multifocal seizures arising from the neocortex have proven refractory to conventional anticonvulsant therapy and newer surgical approaches.[1,2] Even with guidance from modern imaging techniques that allow functional anatomic correlation of seizure onset with surface rendering of the neocortex, surgical treatment of extratemporal epilepsy results in only 36% to 76% of patients being seizure free.[3]

ALTERNATIVES TO PERMANENT RESECTION FOR NEOCORTICAL EPILEPSY

A variety of invasive but nondestructive strategies have been proposed or used to reduce the frequency and severity of neocortical seizures. These strategies include vagal nerve stimulation (VNS), which for the past 15 years has been used for a subset of children and adults with refractory epilepsy.[4,5] Although clinical studies have validated its efficacy, the overall reduction in seizure frequency with VNS was 28% in one randomized controlled trial. Although this reduction represents improved seizure control for some patients, for many others there is insignificant improvement in quality of life.

There is limited experience with several variations of intermittent electrical stimulation for human epilepsy. Recent publications have identified subsets of patients that benefited from intermittent hippocampal or thalamic stimulation.[6] A 2010 prospective trial of anterior thalamic nuclear stimulation reported a seizure reduction of approximately 50%, which was substantial but still insufficient to dramatically improve the quality of their lives.[7]

The most sophisticated intervention currently in clinical trials is a totally implantable closed-loop feedback system for seizure detection and cortical stimulation to terminate focal seizures. This system uses the same electrodes for recording

This work was supported by grants from CURE/DOD (Citizens United for Research in Epilepsy/Department of Defense); NIH, R01-NS042936; and the University of Minnesota Institute for Engineering in Medicine. The authors have nothing to disclose.

[a] Department of Neurosurgery, Washington University, One Children's Place, Suite 4s20, St Louis, MO 63110-1077, USA

[b] Department of Neurology, University of Minnesota Medical School-MMC 486, 420 Delaware Street South East, Minneapolis, MN 55455-0374, USA

* Corresponding author.

E-mail address: smythm@wudosis.wustl.edu

and stimulation with a custom-designed seizure detection algorithm and a device that abruptly terminates seizures by delivering a burst stimulation lasting for about a tenth of a second.[8] This method is being tested at several North American epilepsy centers, yet, to date, its utility seems similar to thalamic stimulation.[9]

An alternative to these strategies is focal cooling, which is a safe nondestructive modality that may provide better seizure control if delivered at the ictal onset. Reports of the effects of direct application of iced saline on the cortical surface during cortical mapping surgery and induced seizures[10,11] have led to interest in developing implantable cooling therapy devices for refractory localizable epilepsies. In the following sections we provide an overview of the historical background, physiology, and animal and human data leading to the development of implantable cooling devices for the treatment of medically refractory epilepsy.

COOLING AND THE BRAIN

Focal brain cooling is an attractive nondestructive strategy to terminate and possibly prevent focal seizures. For several decades, published neurophysiologic studies have illustrated that cooling reduces synaptic transmission in the mammalian brain and that it should be possible to use new engineering technology to deliver focal cooling to superficial and deep brain structures. An 1895 report from Stefani[12] and a 1900 report from Deganello[13] provide the earliest descriptions of the central neurologic effects of focal cooling. A decade later, the German physiologist Trendelenburg began a systematic study of local hypothermia, investigating its effects on brainstem autonomic reflexes and the neocortex.[14] These early investigators concluded that cooling reduced neurologic function at the system level, although none of them had any cellular insights. Throughout the rest of the twentieth century, physiologists continued to use local cooling to investigate cortical and subcortical localization of specific brain functions.

Over the last 50 years, information about the neurobiological effects of cooling has markedly increased. In 1965, Katz and Miledi[15] used intracellular recording at the frog neuromuscular junction to show that cooling prolonged the latency of end plate potentials. The investigators stated that this prolongation likely occurred by desynchronizing acetylcholine release from presynaptic terminals. More recent experiments in mammalian tissue culture and brain slices showed that cooling affects neurotransmission through presynaptic and postsynaptic mechanisms. Two studies published in 1992 and 2001 show that cooling can augment the magnitude of neuronal action potentials and inhibit the sodium/potassium adenosine triphosphatase (ATPase).[16,17] Although the initial ATPase inhibition and concomitant cell depolarization elicited transient hyperexcitability, cooling eventually reduced neuronal excitability. Our own published observations indicate that hypothermia rapidly reduces transmitter release from presynaptic vesicles and suggest that this may be a dominant effect of rapid cooling on central neuronal excitability.[18]

The potential clinical utility of cooling for neurologic disease has been discussed for half a century. Fay[19] began an extensive investigation of brain cooling in 1938. He suggested that systemic hypothermia or local cooling of the brain using chilled fluid circulating through a sealed metal capsule might be an efficacious treatment of head trauma and intractable pain. The investigator also believed that reducing brain temperature could inhibit tumor growth and therefore tried intracranial cooling for inoperable gliomas (**Fig. 1**).

More recent controlled studies have reported the benefits of cooling in patients after acute head trauma or asphyxia.[20–25] The temperature reduction in these recent clinical reports is generally no more than 4°C, which would not be expected to have a very large effect on synaptic transmission. This decrease is also much smaller than the cooling required to terminate severe experimental seizures in rodents.

Physicians have been aware of a causal relationship between elevated temperature and seizures since Hippocrates in 400 BC. Moreover, numerous in vitro and in vivo experimental epilepsy studies have consistently demonstrated that cooling reduces paroxysmal bursting and can diminish or stop seizure activity. Some clinical reports suggest that there is merit in using brain cooling for human seizures as well. At least 5 separate clinical investigations have documented the efficacy of cooling in the therapy for patients with intractable status epilepticus or chronic recurrent seizures. The first study in 6 patients with refractory status epilepticus documented that external cooling (31°C–36°C) stopped seizures in all but one.[26] The second study described 25 patients, aged 8 to 46 years, who had frequent major motor seizures that were poorly controlled by chronic anticonvulsant therapy (**Fig. 2**).[27] While under general anesthesia, these patients were placed in an enclosed chamber and chilled to 29°C with cold air. Bilateral frontal burr holes were opened, and the subarachnoid space or ventricles were irrigated with iced saline, which reduced the cortical surface temperature below 24°C in 21 of the patients. A total volume of 500 to 20,000 mL of

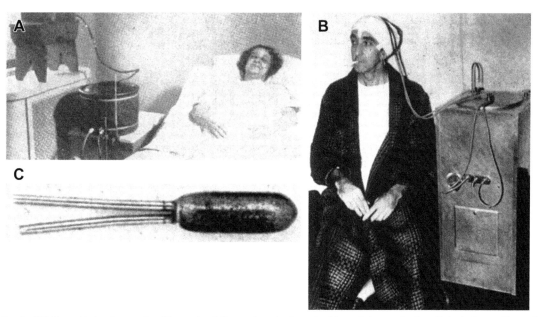

Fig. 1. (*A*) Closed irrigation unit with constant thermal control used with metal capsules for clinical observations of the effect of local refrigeration. (*B*) Patient undergoing focal cooling of resection cavity after a craniotomy for removal of a glioma. (*C*) Irrigation capsule used for intracranial implantation and focal cooling. (*From* Fay T. Early experiences with local and generalized refrigeration of the human brain. J Neurosurg 1959;16:239–60; with permission.)

saline was infused into the patients who were slowly recovered from anesthesia. Of the 15 patients followed up for 1 year, 11 showed a marked reduction in seizure frequency, including 4 who had been seizure free.

The third study documented that vascular cooling to 31°C to 35°C resolved intractable status epilepticus in 4 patients whose seizures persisted despite aggressive intravenous drug therapy that included continuous midazolam or pentobarbital

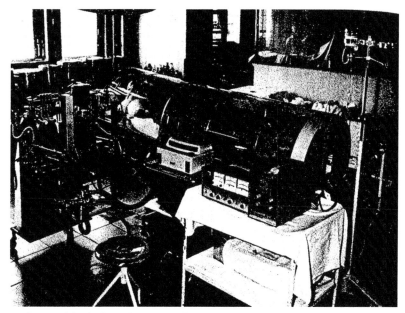

Fig. 2. Apparatus for total body hypothermia with Autohypotherm (Heljestrand, Sweden). (*From* Sourek K, Travnicek V. General and local hypothermia of the brain in the treatment of intractable epilepsy. J Neurosurg 1970;33:253–59; with permission.)

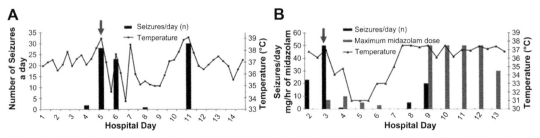

Fig. 3. Relationship between core body temperature and seizure frequency in 2 patients with intractable status epilepticus who were systemically cooled to 34°C and 31°C. Blue arrows indicate onset of cooling. *Panel A*, patient #1; *Panel B*, patient #2.

infusion. All 4 patients had a dramatic reduction in seizures despite the severity of their precooling seizures and the modest degree of cooling (**Fig. 3**).[28] Furthermore, there was clinical and electrographic documentation that cooling influenced the seizures (**Fig. 4**). Two more published studies of human brain cooling during operative neurosurgical mapping confirmed that acutely lowering cortical temperature terminates paroxysmal discharges. In these cases, focal spikes abruptly stopped when iced saline was applied to the neocortex in the operating room.[10,11] Both sets of studies have encouraged the development of more convenient methods of brain cooling for epilepsy.

COOLING METHODOLOGY

Although it would be impractical to design an implanted cooling device for epilepsy therapy based simply on circulating cold water or conventional compressive refrigeration methodology, improvements in thermoelectric devices and their necessary supporting technologies have allowed the reevaluation of cooling as a therapy for some forms of focal epilepsy. Thermoelectric devices use Peltier's 1834 observation that a temperature

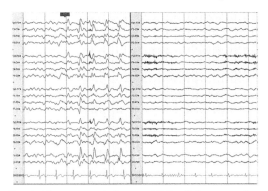

Fig. 4. Electroencephalogram (18 lead) from a patient before cooling (*left panel*) and after cooling (*right panel*). There are very obvious rhythmic seizure discharges seen in the left panel that disappear with cooling (*right panel*).

gradient develops at the junction between 2 dissimilar conductors when an electric current is applied across them. The discovery in the 1920s that synthetic semiconductors were superior to metals as thermoelectric elements hastened progress in this field. Modern semiconductors, typically alloys of bismuth, tellurium, selenium, and antimony, are now used to fabricate small light thermoelectric modules or Peltier devices, which are only a few millimeters in length and width and about 1.5 mm thick (**Fig. 5**A).[29] In these modules, pairs of N- and P-type semiconductors are connected between 2 ceramic plates so that they are electrically in series and thermally in parallel. The latest thermoelectric devices are fabricated with thin film, which was developed for the microelectronics industry, and can be less than 200 μm thick. These devices have up to 10 times the heat pumping capability of conventional devices, making them ideal for medical devices (see **Fig. 5**B).

Thermoelectric devices can generate temperature differentials of 70°C, but, for this to result in cooling, heat must be efficiently removed from the warm side. For most of our work, we attach the warm side of the device to a copper rod, which removes heat and acts as a convenient holder for a manipulator. When our work advances to the point of requiring internal heat dissipation, we use heat pipes that have been designed to efficiently transfer heat to highly vascularized areas of the skull or dura.

RESULTS USING EPILEPSY ANIMAL MODELS

In 1999, we learned about the attractive features of commercially available thermoelectric devices and thus began experiments to determine whether they could terminate acute seizures.[30] After we found that we could use cooling to stop seizurelike events in rat brain slices, we looked for an in vivo effect of cooling on focal cortical seizures. We discovered that we could reliably induce focal seizures in halothane-anesthetized rats by injecting a tiny volume of 4-aminopyridine (4-AP) solution 0.5 mm below the pial surface of the motor

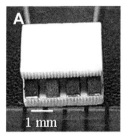
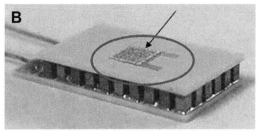

Fig. 5. (*A*) Conventional thermoelectric cooling device of about 4 × 4 mm². Individual semiconductors and ceramic wafers are easily seen. (*B*) On top of another conventional thermoelectric cooler (*within circle*) is a new ultrathin thermoelectric cooler that could be the basis for an implantable device. (*Courtesy of* Nextreme Thermal Solutions, Durham, NC, USA; with permission.)

cortex using a micropipette. Within 20 minutes, the animals developed recurrent focal seizures and continued to have electrographic seizures for approximately 2 hours. Untreated seizures lasted between 60 and 80 seconds. We then maneuvered a thermoelectric device to directly contact the neocortex immediately above the injection site and at seizure onset and activated cooling to 20°C. This process reduced seizure duration to approximately 7 seconds (**Figs. 6** and **7**).[31] We believed that this rapid effect was because of the local cooling because the thermoelectric device did not influence seizure duration if it was not in direct contact with the cortical surface (see **Figs. 6**B and **7**). In this case, there was a progressive decrease in seizure duration when we cooled between 26°C and 22°C.

After completing our initial cooling experiments, we developed a frequency-based seizure detection algorithm for the 4-AP seizures, which allowed us to use a closed-loop system to abort seizures.[32] To minimize false-positives, we set a relatively high threshold before cooling was activated. In these circumstances, our closed-loop system was as effective in terminating seizures as manual activation. Had we decided to accept more false-positives, we could have initiated more rapid cooling and further reduced seizure duration.

Since that time, we investigated other important aspects of cooling for focal seizures. In one case,

we used a small thermocouple inserted into a 30-gauge needle to map the cortex below our thermoelectric device, which showed that cooling extends only about 4 mm below the surface. This finding demonstrated that the cooling effect should be localized to just a small region of neocortex below the pia.[32]

A series of experiments replicated and extended our observation that cooling attenuates experimental epilepsy. In kindled rat hippocampal seizures, seizure severity and afterdischarge duration were reduced with cooling between 23°C and 26°C and with saline flowing through thin copper tubing next to the dorsal hippocampus (**Fig. 8**).[33] Another laboratory using Peltier devices almost identical to those used in our work showed that cortical excitability triggered by local injection of kainic acid was reduced by focal cooling.[34] This group then showed that they could cool deep into the rat hippocampus by attaching an insulated needle to a Peltier device held away from the brain surface.[35]

Ongoing experiments are evaluating the efficacy of focal cooling on antiepileptogenesis and anti-ictogenesis in a rodent model of pharmacoresistant posttraumatic epilepsy: the fluid percussion injury model (CURE/DOD USAMRMC 05154001.5 and 08149006) (**Fig. 9**).[36–38] We are currently preparing a comprehensive manuscript detailing substantial data confirming the efficacy of a double-blinded

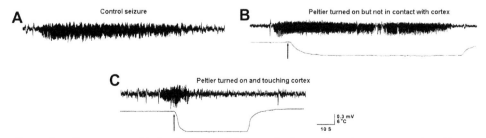

Fig. 6. Effects of cooling on rats with focal seizures. (*A*) Control seizure. The seizures were reduced by more than 90% in duration (*C*). There was no effect of cooling close to the seizure focus if the cooling device did not make direct contact (*B*). (*From* Yang XF, Rothman SM. Focal cooling rapidly terminates experimental neocortical seizures. Annals of Neurology 2001;49:721–26; with permission.)

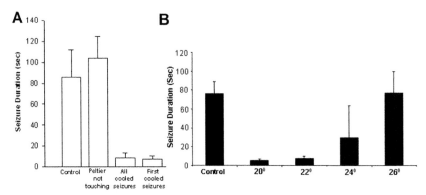

Fig. 7. Effects of cooling on seizure durations in rats. (*A*) Seizure durations are reduced, on average, by 90%. The effect of cooling is the same when it is repeated on subsequent seizures as on the first seizure. (*B*) There is fairly steep temperature dependence of the 4-AP–induced seizures. Above 26°C, the durations of these seizures are the same as control, but, between 20 and 24°C, they shorten dramatically. (*From* Yang XF, Rothman SM. Focal cooling rapidly terminates experimental neocortical seizures. Ann Neurol 2001;49:721–26; with permission.)

randomized trial of focal cortical cooling using this model.

A limited set of unpublished observations on a single monkey verified that our thermoelectric device is capable of inhibiting function in the primate neocortex. When our thermoelectric device was placed in direct contact with the pia on the surface of the hand region of the precentral gyrus, there was a consistent reversible impairment in skilled finger movements associated with a reduction in surface temperature. This occurrence indicates that the small thermoelectric devices have sufficient power to cool primate cortex. Of note, even with cooling to 10°C, the impairment was not instantaneous and did not completely paralyze hand movements (S. Rothman, MD, unpublished data, 2005).

COOLING-INDUCED CORTICAL INJURY

Recent work has explored the possibility of brain damage induced by local cooling. Thus far, we have not seen any evidence that cooling as low as 5°C, far below our target temperature for clinical use, for 2 hours produces neuronal loss or activates apoptotic pathways (**Figs. 10–12**).[39] Although there is minimal gliosis close to the region of cortical contact with the Peltier, it is similar to the response provoked by any foreign body and cannot be attributed to cooling. When brain slices obtained from transgenic mice expressing the green fluorescent protein were cooled to 5°C, there was transient, but completely reversible, blebbing of dendrite shafts and loss of spines. Blebbing is probably secondary to ion pump inhibition because other investigators

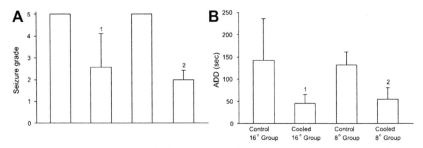

Fig. 8. Effect of cooling on seizure grade and afterdischarge duration (ADD). (*A*) Cooling with 16°C and 8°C coolants significantly reduced seizure grade from corresponding controls (1, 2; *P*<.001 analysis of variance [ANOVA] followed by Student-Newman-Keuls method). No significant difference in seizure score was found between the 2 coolant temperatures (*P* = .28). No error bars are present for seizure grade in controls because all seizures, by our criteria, were grade 5 before initiating cooling. (*B*) Cooling with 16°C and 8°C coolants significantly reduced ADD from corresponding controls (1, 2; *P*<.005 ANOVA followed by Student-Newman-Keuls method). No significant difference in ADD was found between the coolant temperatures (*P* = .077). (*From* Burton JM, Peebles GA, Binder DK, et al. Transcortical cooling inhibits hippocampal-kindled seizures in the rat. Epilepsia 2005;46(12):1881–7; with permission.)

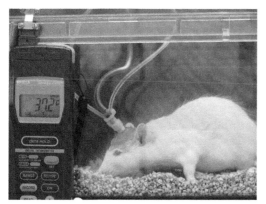

Fig. 9. Neocortical cooling implant in adult rat consisting of a stainless steel cooling element on the frontal lobe capable of circulating coolant of any desired temperature. Thermocouple reading indicates the non-cooled brain temperature, 37.2°C. 5 Channel EEG electrode wires are protected from by the coiled sheath. Dental acrylic secures the cooling element, EEG electrodes and thermocouple.

made similar observations after treating brain slices with sodium/potassium ATPase inhibitors.[40] We also failed to observe any neuronal loss in cat neocortex after 7 to 10 months of intermittent cooling during neurophysiologic experiments. Thus, we are optimistic that the effect of cooling will be exquisitely focal and well tolerated.

HEAT DISSIPATION

To move ahead with the design of a fully implantable cooling device for human focal epilepsy, we have begun to address the problem of heat dissipation from the warm side of thermoelectric devices. Although a copper rod has worked well for experiments in anesthetized or immobilized animals, a more compact device is required to transfer heat from a clinical device. There is extensive literature describing heat pipes, which rapidly equilibrate temperature across a distance by allowing a liquid to alternately evaporate and recondense under reduced atmospheric pressure within a hollow, evacuated, wicked tube. Our engineering colleagues have designed a thin malleable laminar heat pipe composed of outer layers of copper foil and an inner layer of sintered copper columns sandwiched between 2 layers of sintered copper.[41] The charging fluid is water, which flows between the copper columns. The pipe should be capable of transferring sufficient heat from a thermoelectric device so that a cold side temperature of 20°C could be maintained without heating the adjacent brain more than 38°C. We envision positioning a similar heat pipe between the warm side of a thermoelectric device and the dura, skull, or scalp, so that heat can be efficiently transferred to one of these highly vascular compartments for internal heat dissipation.

THE PATH TO CLINICAL COOLING DEVICES

The most critical question at this time is regarding the degree of cooling required to terminate or prevent human focal seizures. It is unlikely that current animal models will help us to answer this question. Although the fluid percussion injury model is promising, there is no validated rodent model of chronic focal epilepsy that reliably reproduces the human condition. The 4-AP model, which we have used in our studies, is much more severe than even the most refractory human epilepsy.[31] These rats typically have 60- to 80-minute seizures every 2 to 3 minutes, which is an unrealistically high frequency for almost all human epilepsies. We already know that these seizures are relatively unresponsive to parenteral diazepam at doses that eliminate status epilepticus in other rat models. Therefore, it seems likely that these rodent focal seizures require a much larger temperature reduction than human seizures.

Because the required degree of cooling governs the current that is required to power the thermoelectric device, it is critical to determine the temperature sensitivity of human focal epilepsy. Moreover, the degree of cooling determines the amount of heat that has to be dissipated to the vasculature or dura through a heat pipe. To investigate this issue, we fabricated a cooling device that uses cold saline rather than a thermoelectric device. The device combines a conventional Silastic grid used for invasive monitoring and a bladder through which cold saline flows.

GRID/COOLING BLADDER RESULTS: IN VIVO TESTS

With approval from the University of Minnesota's Institutional Animal Care and Use Committee, we were able to verify that we could safely and effectively cool the neocortex in 2 dogs. To accomplish this, each dog was placed under general anesthesia and the bone flap was removed, exposing the cortex. The standard small grid (**Fig. 13**A) was first inserted over the neocortex, and control electroencephalographic (EEG) result was sampled. The grid was then replaced with the small grid/cooling bladder (see **Fig. 13**B), which was connected to a standard clinical peristaltic pump. The tubing flowed through a cooling bath placed within 2 ft of the head, so that there was minimal temperature drop between the cooling bath and the grid/cooling bladder. Standard thermocouples were

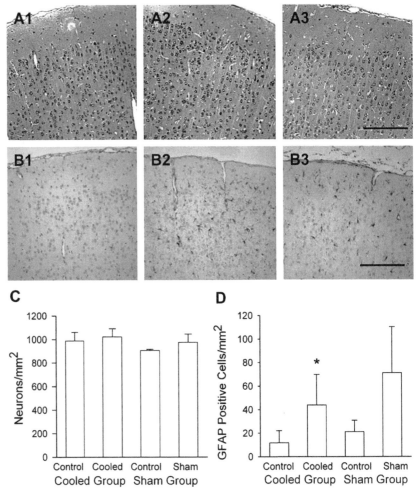

Fig. 10. Effects of cooling on neocortical neurons and glia. (A) Cresyl violet staining reveals no diffe[r]
between control neocortex (A1), contralateral cortex in direct contact with thermoelectric device at 5[°]
then recovered for 2 days (A2), and cortex in contact with device that was not turned on (A3). (B) Glial fi[brillary]
acidic protein (GFAP) staining of control neocortex (B1) shows fewer positive cells than either cooled cort[ex]
or cortex placed in contact with inactive thermoelectric device (B3). (C) Counts revealed no difference in n[eurons]
in cortex from cooled and sham-operated controls ($P = .2$ by analysis of variance; N = 5 for control and [cooled]
cortex and 3 for sham controls). (D) There was a difference between cooled and control cortex in the num[ber of]
GFAP-positive cells in the cohort of 5 animals whose cortical temperature was reduced to 5°C ($*P = .04$ by [paired]
t test compared with control side). However, an identical effect of touching neocortex without cooling wa[s seen]
in the sham surgery group. (Calibration in A3 and B3, 200 μm.) (From Yang XF, Kennedy BR, Lomber SG[, et al.]
Cooling produces minimal neuropathology in neocortex and hippocampus. Neurobiol Dis 2006;23:637–4[8; with]
permission.)

used to measure the temperature within the bladder and at the interface between the bladder and neocortex. The electrodes on the grid were connected to a standard clinical EEG amplifier, and the output was archived on a laptop computer.

The grid/cooling bladder was perfused with saline at room temperature, 10°C, and 0°C at 10 and 20 mL/min. We found that we could cool the brain/cooling bladder interface to less than 20°C when we used saline chilled to 0°C. We saw no deterioration in the quality of the EEG recording

during the perfusion and cooling. We d[id]
control depth of anesthesia accurately eno[ugh to]
comment on physiologic effects of cooli[ng on]
EEG but did not detect any deterioration [in the]
quality of the EEG signal while we perfus[ed the]
grid/cooling bladder (see **Fig. 13**). **Fig. 14**
the temperature recorded from inside the b[ladder]
and at the brain/cooling bladder interface [when]
the saline was only cooled to 10°C and the [perfu-]
sion rate was 10 mL/min. We were still able t[o cool]
the brain surface to less than 27°C. Neoc[ortical]

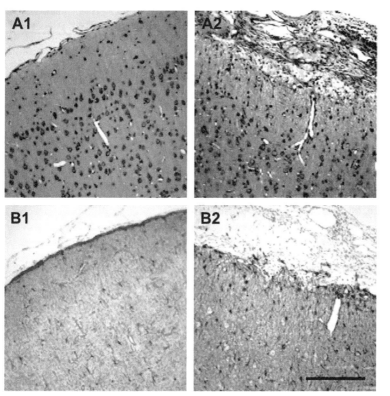

Fig. 11. Effect of cooling to 3°C on cat neocortex. (A) Cresyl violet staining shows little difference in neurons between control (A1) and cooled (A2) cortex, except in the superficial layer immediately adjacent to the thickened arachnoid. (B) There are more glial fibrillary acidic protein–stained cells in cooled (B2) than control (B1) neocortex. Arachnoid thickening is evident in the cooled cortex, but underlying brain is not damaged. (Calibration in B2, 20 μm.) (*From* Yang XF, Kennedy BR, Lomber SG, et al. Cooling produces minimal neuropathology in neocortex and hippocampus. Neurobiol Dis 2006;23:637–43; with permission.)

biopsy results obtained from both study dogs showed no pathologic changes beyond expected from insertion of standard invasive EEG monitoring grids.

Since validating the grid/cooling bladder technology in the dogs, a similar device has been tested intraoperatively in anesthetized patients at Washington University while measuring temperatures

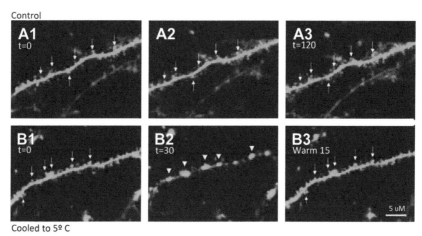

Fig. 12. Effect of cooling on mouse hippocampal slices, imaged with 2-photon microscopy. (A) Control slice from mouse expressing green fluorescent protein has multiple spines readily identified in a single section from a Z-stack (*arrows, A1*). At 32° C, after 60 and 120 minutes (A2 and A3, respectively), the same spines are still evident. (B) Cooling the bath perfusion fluid to 5°C reversibly alters dendritic anatomy. Spines are easily seen in control slice (*arrows, B1*). After 30 minutes, there is beading of the dendritic shaft (*arrowheads*), but some spines are still present (B2). After 15 minutes of rewarming to 32° C, the beading has disappeared and the spines that were initially present are again evident (B3). (Calibration in B3, 5 μm.) (*From* Yang XF, Kennedy BR, Lomber SG, et al. Cooling produces minimal neuropathology in neocortex and hippocampus. Neurobiol Dis 2006;23: 637–43; with permission.)

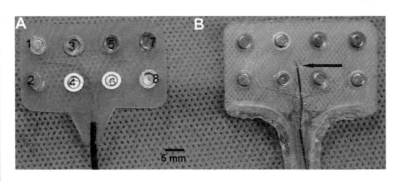

Fig. 13. (A) Standard com cial 4 × 2 electrode gr invasive intracranial ma of focal epileptic disch The green wires in the connect to the blue which is routed to an e encephalographic amplif Modified grid, similar t except that it has anothe of Silastic fastened a periphery, creating a wate bladder. Inflow and o tubing connect into the bladder at the bottom. The black arrow points to a thermocouple that records tempe within the bladder. This type of grid was used in the canine experiments described. The grids are manufactu PMT (Chanhassen, MN, USA); www.pmtcorp.com.

at the grid/brain interface and at depths of 5, 10, and 15 mm in the cortex during simultaneous electrocorticography. The bladder was perfused with sterile iced saline, and temperatures were continuously monitored. We found that we could lower the cortical surface temperature to 26°C with confirmed effective stable cooling to 10 mm (**Fig. 15**, Matthew Smyth, MD, unpublished data, 2010). Our next study will entail temporary implantation of the cooling bladder/grid in patients with focal epilepsy during invasive monitoring, before surgical resection. It would permit determination of the degree of cooling required to stop paroxysmal activity (spikes and high-frequency oscillations) and seizures without having to cope with internal heat dissipation. Once the cooling parameters (and thus power requirements) have been better defined, it will be possible to rationally

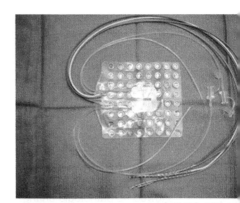

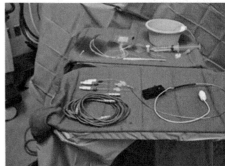

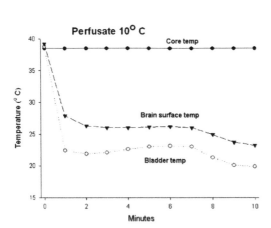

Fig. 14. Results of testing cooling grid (see **Fig. 13**B) in dogs. When chilled saline (10°C) perfused the bladder at 10 ml/min, the internal temperature of the bladder decreased and the temperature at the interface between the cortex and grid decreased from 25°C to 26°C. The core temperature of the dog remained at 38°C.

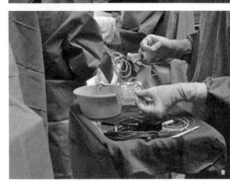

Fig. 15. Testing 8 × 8 cooling bladder/grid in a p at St Louis Children's Hospital before resecti epilepsy.

design a fully implantable device using thermoelectric technology.

COOLING DEVICE PROTOTYPES AND CONCEPTS
Addressing Mesial Temporal Lobe Epilepsy

In many patients with temporal lobe epilepsy, temporal lobectomy and its variations result in excellent outcomes.[42–44] However, resection of mesial temporal structures does carry the risk of irreversible visual, neurocognitive, and memory deficits.[45–48] Placing a focal cooling probe stereotactically into the amygdala-hippocampal formation may prove to be a viable treatment of mesial temporal sclerosis without subjecting patients to the neuropsychological deficits of temporal resection. Such a device concept is depicted in **Fig. 16**. A semirigid heat pipe, partially insulated, allows near-instantaneous cooling of the deep portion when cooling is applied to the extracranial end of the heat pipe. A separate battery/computer module provides the power source for the Peltier component in contact with the heat pipe and allows for responsive cooling with seizure detection/prediction algorithms or chronic continuous/intermittent cooling of the deep mesial structures. A subgaleal or epidural baffle provides a large surface area for heat dissipation adjacent to the vascularized dura or scalp. The usefulness of an implantable electrically driven brain cooling device

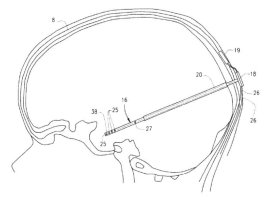

Fig. 16. Depth cooling device concept. A partially insulated (20) heat pipe (16) is implanted stereotactically into amygdalohippocampal formation through the skull (8). A thermocouple (38) and electrodes (25) are integrated into the noninsulated deep portion of the heat pipe. A Peltier-based cooling element (18) contacts the superficial portion of the heat pipe, with a subgaleal heat sink (19) attached via another flexible heat pipe to the warm side of the Peltier. Wires for power supply and electrode recording (26) run subcutaneously to a separate power supply/computer controller.[50]

may well extend beyond therapy for pharmacoresistant epilepsy. Implantable cooling probes or plates may provide a superior alternative to methods that are currently used in functional neurosurgery, such as ablative procedures for pain and movement disorders, and may well be more efficacious than deep brain stimulation for reversibly deactivating or modulating activity in deep structures. Cooling for these clinical problems requires prolonged activation of a Peltier device, so improvements in battery technology are required before this area of research can proceed.

Addressing Neocortical Epilepsy

Although current techniques of seizure localization and resection of epileptogenic tissue frequently result in seizure freedom, often the ictal zone is poorly localized or involves eloquent cortex. Focal cortical surface cooling may provide a means of seizure control by recalibrating the ictal threshold without affecting normal cortical function. We have yet to determine the critical temperatures necessary for anticonvulsant efficacy without affecting function but suspect that the critical temperature is well above those that cause functional neural suppression. The current grid prototypes undergoing testing use fluid circulation for cooling and heat dissipation, but a fully implantable device incorporates a thermocouple array with electrocorticographic electrodes and a battery/computer module serving as a power source and controller (**Fig. 17**). An additional capability of an implantable brain cooling system is the ability to perform a temporary resection of a region of cortex. Current brain mapping techniques (intraoperative and postoperative with subdural grid arrays) rely on electrical stimulation to activate regions (mapping primary motor cortex) or disrupt normal function (speech arrest, anomia in language mapping). Reversibly inactivating a region of the cortex allows the evaluation of clinical deficits before committing to a permanent resection. Cooling technology could be used in intraoperative and invasive bedside brain mapping as an adjunct to resections for epilepsy and neoplastic disorders. The group in Iowa has used a handheld cooling device for intraoperative testing of functional deactivation of eloquent cortex, including Broca area, with interesting results.[49]

CRITICISMS

We recognize that there are clear obstacles and objections to focal cooling for human seizures. First, because of convolutions in the human brain, approximately two-thirds of the neocortex is

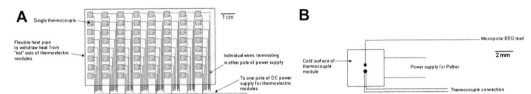

Fig. 17. Cooling electrocorticographic grid for neocortical epilepsy. (*A*) Each individual thermoelectric module can be independently activated. All are in contact with a thin bendable heat pipe that is in direct physical contact with the hot side. There are also a silver microelectrode and miniature thermocouple on the surface of each thermoelectric module to monitor epidural EEG changes and temperature, respectively. (*B*) Enlarged surface of single thermoelectric module, showing power connection, monopolar EEG monitoring lead, and thermocouple connectors.

buried in sulci, making it inaccessible to surface cooling. However, it should still be possible to cool portions of the substantial area of exposed cortex that are responsible for generating seizures. In addition, cooling the superficial lip of cortical sulci may block the spread of seizures arising deeper within the sulci. It should even be feasible to connect thin flexible heat pipes to thermoelectric devices to cool structures deeper in the brain (see **Fig. 16**).[41,50] Second, cooling may be as disruptive to normal brain function as some seizures are. We are optimistic that there is a temperature range that separates seizure control from disruption of normal cortical function. Supporting this hope are study results from Bakken and colleagues[49] showing that cooling below 10°C over eloquent cortex did not produce a complete anomia or non-fluent aphasia. Third, although we are concerned that the power required for thermoelectric devices is quite high, the short duty cycle may allow these devices to operate for long periods without re-charge or replacement. Moreover, battery life improvements and thin film thermoelectric design should make it possible to generate more efficient devices soon. Last, although there is presently no fully validated algorithm for human seizure detection or prediction, an adequate detection algorithm has already been implemented in the responsive stimulation device now in clinical trials.[51] Moreover, prediction algorithms using an implanted grid are in human trials in Australia (NCT01043406; www.neurovista.com). We would ultimately be able to cool responsively using either system to activate an implanted thermoelectric module.

We anticipate that we will make substantial progress over the next 5 years toward the design and implementation of focal brain cooling devices for the control of refractory focal epilepsy. New data from an even more realistic animal model of human epilepsy (currently unpublished) demonstrate very promising antiepileptogenic and anti-epileptic efficacies of focal cooling.[36–38] We are now at a critical inflection point, having moved from bench-top experiments and animal models to actual clinical prototype design and testing in humans. Progressive advancements in biotechnology that involve miniaturization, battery technology, seizure detection/prediction algorithms, and thin film thermoelectric design may very well intersect with ongoing and planned clinical trials of focal cooling in humans. This intersection could lead to the production of small effective devices for focally cooling a variety of regions of the human brain to control refractory epilepsy while preserving neurologic function.

ACKNOWLEDGMENTS

The authors wish to express their appreciation for their ongoing collaborative investigations of cortical cooling for epilepsy with Raimondo D'Ambrosio, PhD (Department of Neurosurgery, University of Washington, Seattle), and John Miller, MD, PhD (Department of Neurosurgery, University of Washington, Seattle).

REFERENCES

1. O'Brien TJ, So EL, Mullan BP, et al. Subtraction peri-ictal SPECT is predictive of extratemporal epilepsy surgery outcome. Neurology 2000;55(11):1668–77.
2. Cascino GD. Surgical treatment for extratemporal epilepsy. Curr Treat Options Neurol 2004;6(3):257–62.
3. Olivier A. Surgery of extratemporal epilepsy. Baltimore (MD): Williams & Wilkins; 1997.
4. Murphy JV. Left vagal nerve stimulation in children with medically refractory epilepsy. The Pediatric VNS Study Group. J Pediatr 1999;134(5):563–6.
5. Nakken KO, Henriksen O, Roste GK, et al. Vagal nerve stimulation—the Norwegian experience. Seizure 2003;12(1):37–41.
6. Lesser RP, Theodore WH. If not pharmacology, maybe physics. Neurology 2006;66(10):1468–9.

7. Fisher R, Salanova V, Witt T, et al. Electrical stimulation of the anterior nucleus of thalamus for treatment of refractory epilepsy. Epilepsia 2010;51(5):899–908.

8. Morrell M. Brain stimulation for epilepsy: can scheduled or responsive neurostimulation stop seizures? Curr Opin Neurol 2006;19(2):164–8.

9. Morrell M. Results of a multicenter double blinded randomized controlled pivotal investigation of the RNS™ System for treatment of intractable partial epilepsy in adults, vol. 1. Boston: American Epilepsy Society; 2009. p. 102.

10. Sartorius CJ, Berger MS. Rapid termination of intra-operative stimulation-evoked seizures with application of cold Ringer's lactate to the cortex. Technical note. J Neurosurg 1998;88(2):349–51.

11. Karkar KM, Garcia PA, Bateman LM, et al. Focal cooling suppresses spontaneous epileptiform activity without changing the cortical motor threshold. Epilepsia 2002;43(8):932–5.

12. Stefani A. De l'action de la temperature sur les centres bulbaires du coeur et des vaisseaux. Arch Ital Biol 1895;24:424–37.

13. Deganello U. Action de la temperature sur le centre bulbaire inhibiteur du coeur et sur le centre bulbaire vaso-constricteur. Arch Ital Biol 1900;33:186–8 [in French].

14. Brooks V. Study of brain function by local, reversible cooling. Rev Physiol Biochem Pharmacol 1983;95: 1–109.

15. Katz B, Miledi R. The effect of temperature on the synaptic delay at the neuromuscular junction. J Physiol 1965;181(3):656–70.

16. Voiculescu V, Voinescu I. Effect of hypothermia on focal experimental seizures. Rom J Neurol Psychiatry 1992;30(4):237–42.

17. Aihara H, Okada Y, Tamaki N. The effects of cooling and rewarming on the neuronal activity of pyramidal neurons in guinea pig hippocampal slices. Brain Res 2001;893(1–2):36–45.

18. Yang XF, Ouyang Y, Kennedy BR, et al. Cooling blocks rat hippocampal neurotransmission by a presynaptic mechanism: observations using 2-photon microscopy. J Physiol 2005;567(Pt 1):215–24.

19. Fay T. Early experiences with local and generalized refrigeration of the human brain. J Neurosurg 1959; 16(3):239–59 [discussion: 259–60].

20. Azzopardi D, Robertson NJ, Cowan FM, et al. Pilot study of treatment with whole body hypothermia for neonatal encephalopathy. Pediatrics 2000; 106(4):684–94.

21. Edwards AD, Wyatt JS, Thoresen M. Treatment of hypoxic-ischaemic brain damage by moderate hypothermia. Arch Dis Child Fetal Neonatal Ed 1998; 78(2):F85–8.

22. Inder TE, Hunt RW, Morley CJ, et al. Randomized trial of systemic hypothermia selectively protects the cortex on MRI in term hypoxic-ischemic encephalopathy. J Pediatr 2004;145(6):835–7.

23. Laptook AR, Corbett RJ, Sterett R, et al. Modest hypothermia provides partial neuroprotection when used for immediate resuscitation after brain ischemia. Pediatr Res 1997;42(1):17–23.

24. Shankaran S, Laptook AR, Ehrenkranz RA, et al. Whole-body hypothermia for neonates with hypoxic-ischemic encephalopathy. N Engl J Med 2005; 353(15):1574–84.

25. Walpoth BH, Walpoth-Aslan BN, Mattle HP, et al. Outcome of survivors of accidental deep hypothermia and circulatory arrest treated with extracorporeal blood warming. N Engl J Med 1997; 337(21):1500–5.

26. Vastola EF, Homan R, Rosen A. Inhibition of focal seizures by moderate hypothermia. A clinical and experimental study. Arch Neurol 1969;20(4):430–9.

27. Sourek K, Travnicek V. General and local hypothermia of the brain in the treatment of intractable epilepsy. J Neurosurg 1970;33(3):253–9.

28. Corry JJ, Dhar R, Murphy T, et al. Hypothermia for refractory status epilepticus. Neurocrit Care 2008; 9(2):189–97.

29. Sales BC. Thermoelectric materials. Smaller is cooler. Science 2002;295(5558):1248–9.

30. Hill MW, Wong M, Amarakone A, et al. Rapid cooling aborts seizure-like activity in rodent hippocampal-entorhinal slices. Epilepsia 2000; 41(10):1241–8.

31. Yang XF, Rothman SM. Focal cooling rapidly terminates experimental neocortical seizures. Ann Neurol 2001;49(6):721–6.

32. Yang XF, Duffy DW, Morley RE, et al. Neocortical seizure termination by focal cooling: temperature dependence and automated seizure detection. Epilepsia 2002;43(3):240–5.

33. Burton JM, Peebles GA, Binder DK, et al. Transcortical cooling inhibits hippocampal-kindled seizures in the rat. Epilepsia 2005;46(12):1881–7.

34. Imoto H, Fujii M, Uchiyama J, et al. Use of a Peltier chip with a newly devised local brain-cooling system for neocortical seizures in the rat. Technical note. J Neurosurg 2006;104(1):150–6.

35. Tanaka N, Fujii M, Imoto H, et al. Effective suppression of hippocampal seizures in rats by direct hippocampal cooling with a Peltier chip. J Neurosurg 2008;108(4):791–7.

36. D'Ambrosio R, Fairbanks JP, Fender JS, et al. Post-traumatic epilepsy following fluid percussion injury in the rat. Brain 2004;127:304–14.

37. D'Ambrosio R, Fender JS, Fairbanks JP, et al. Progression from frontal-parietal to mesial-temporal epilepsy after fluid percussion injury in the rat. Brain 2005;128:174–88.

38. Eastman CL, Verley DR, Fender JS, et al. ECoG studies of valproate, carbamazepine and halothane

in frontal-lobe epilepsy induced by head injury in the rat. Exp Neurol 2010;224:369–88.

39. Yang XF, Kennedy BR, Lomber SG, et al. Cooling produces minimal neuropathology in neocortex and hippocampus. Neurobiol Dis 2006;23(3):637–43.

40. Kirov SA, Petrak LJ, Fiala JC, et al. Dendritic spines disappear with chilling but proliferate excessively upon rewarming of mature hippocampus. Neuroscience 2004;127(1):69–80.

41. Hilderbrand JK, Peterson GP, Rothman SM. Development of a phase change heat spreader to enable focal cooling as a treatment for intractable neocortical epilepsy. Heat Transfer Engineering 2007;28:282–91.

42. Wiebe S, Blume WT, Girvin JP, et al. A randomized, controlled trial of surgery for temporal-lobe epilepsy. N Engl J Med 2001;345(5):311–8.

43. Spencer DD, Spencer SS, Mattson RH, et al. Access to the posterior medial temporal lobe structures in the surgical treatment of temporal lobe epilepsy. Neurosurgery 1984;15(5):667–71.

44. Smyth MD, Limbrick DD Jr, Ojemann JG, et al. Outcome following surgery for temporal lobe epilepsy with hippocampal involvement in preadolescent children: emphasis on mesial temporal sclerosis. J Neurosurg 2007;106(Suppl 3):205–10.

45. Yam D, Nicolle D, Steven DA, et al. Visual field deficits following anterior temporal lobectomy: long-term follow-up and prognostic implications. Epilepsia 2010;51(6):1018–23.

46. Pillon B, Bazin B, Deweer B, et al. Specificity of memory deficits after right or left temporal lobectomy. Cortex 1999;35(4):561–71.

47. Huxlin KR, Merigan WH. Deficits in complex visual perception following unilateral temporal lobectomy. J Cogn Neurosci 1998;10(3):395–407.

48. Feigenbaum JD, Polkey CE, Morris RG. Deficits in spatial working memory after unilateral temporal lobectomy in man. Neuropsychologia 1996;34(3):163–76.

49. Bakken HE, Kawasaki H, Oya H, et al. A device for cooling localized regions of human cerebral cortex. Technical note. J Neurosurg 2003;99(3):604–8.

50. Smyth MD. Depth Cooling Implant System. US Patent 12/164,857, Filed June 30, 2008, published January 1, 2009. Assignee: Washington University in St. Louis.

51. Snyder DE, Echauz J, Grimes DB, et al. The statistics of a practical seizure warning system. J Neural Eng 2008;5(4):392–401.

Index

Neurosurg Clin N Am 22 (2011) 547–549
doi:10.1016/S1042-3680(11)00092-1
1042-3680/11/$ – see front matter

United States Postal Service

Statement of Ownership, Management, and Circulation
(All Periodicals Publications Except Requestor Publications)

1. Publication Title
Neurosurgery Clinics of North America

2. Publication Number
0 1 3 - 1 2 4

3. Filing Date
9/16/11

4. Issue Frequency
Jan, Apr, Jul, Oct

5. Number of Issues Published Annually
4

6. Annual Subscription Price
$317.00

7. Complete Mailing Address of Known Office of Publication (Not printer) (Street, city, county, state, and ZIP+4®)
Elsevier Inc.
360 Park Avenue South
New York, NY 10010-1710

Contact Person
Amy S.Beacham

Telephone (Include area code)
215-239-3687

8. Complete Mailing Address of Headquarters or General Business Office of Publisher (Not printer)
Elsevier Inc., 360 Park Avenue South, New York, NY 10010-1710

9. Full Names and Complete Mailing Addresses of Publisher, Editor, and Managing Editor (Do not leave blank)

Publisher (Name and complete mailing address)
Kim Murphy, Elsevier, Inc., 1600 John F. Kennedy Blvd. Suite 1800, Philadelphia, PA 19103-2899

Editor (Name and complete mailing address)
Jessica McCool, Elsevier, Inc., 1600 John F. Kennedy Blvd. Suite 1800, Philadelphia, PA 19103-2899

Managing Editor (Name and complete mailing address)
Barbara Cohen-Kligerman, Elsevier, Inc., 1600 John F. Kennedy Blvd. Suite 1800, Philadelphia, PA 19103-2899

10. Owner (Do not leave blank. If the publication is owned by a corporation, give the name and address of the corporation immediately followed by the names and addresses of all stockholders owning or holding 1 percent or more of the total amount of stock. If not owned by a corporation, give the names and addresses of the individual owners. If owned by a partnership or other unincorporated firm, give its name and address as well as those of each individual owner. If the publication is published by a nonprofit organization, give its name and address.)

Full Name	Complete Mailing Address
Wholly owned subsidiary of	4520 East-West Highway
Reed/Elsevier, US holdings	Bethesda, MD 20814

11. Known Bondholders, Mortgagees, and Other Security Holders Owning or Holding 1 Percent or More of Total Amount of Bonds, Mortgages, or Other Securities. If none, check box ☐ None

Full Name	Complete Mailing Address
N/A	

12. Tax Status (For completion by nonprofit organizations authorized to mail at nonprofit rates) (Check one)
The purpose, function, and nonprofit status of this organization and the exempt status for federal income tax purposes:
☐ Has Not Changed During Preceding 12 Months
☐ Has Changed During Preceding 12 Months (Publisher must submit explanation of change with this statement)

PS Form 3526, September 2007 (Page 1 of 3 (Instructions Page 3)) PSN 7530-01-000-9931 **PRIVACY NOTICE**: See our Privacy policy in www.usps.com

---

13. Publication Title
Neurosurgery Clinics of North America

14. Issue Date for Circulation Data Below
April 2011

15. Extent and Nature of Circulation

			Average No. Copies Each Issue During Preceding 12 Months	No. Copies of Single Issue Published Nearest to Filing Date
a. Total Number of Copies (Net press run)			1035	850
b. Paid Circulation (By Mail and Outside the Mail)	(1)	Mailed Outside-County Paid Subscriptions Stated on PS Form 3541. (Include paid distribution above nominal rate, advertiser's proof copies, and exchange copies)	353	310
	(2)	Mailed In-County Paid Subscriptions Stated on PS Form 3541 (Include paid distribution above nominal rate, advertiser's proof copies, and exchange copies)		
	(3)	Paid Distribution Outside the Mails Including Sales Through Dealers and Carriers, Street Vendors, Counter Sales, and Other Paid Distribution Outside USPS®	165	95
	(4)	Paid Distribution by Other Classes Mailed Through the USPS (e.g. First-Class Mail®)		
c. Total Paid Distribution (Sum of 15b (1), (2), (3), and (4))		▲	518	405
d. Free or Nominal Rate Distribution (By Mail and Outside the Mail)	(1)	Free or Nominal Rate Outside-County Copies Included on PS Form 3541	49	55
	(2)	Free or Nominal Rate In-County Copies Included on PS Form 3541		
	(3)	Free or Nominal Rate Copies Mailed at Other Classes Through the USPS (e.g. First-Class Mail)		
	(4)	Free or Nominal Rate Distribution Outside the Mail (Carriers or other means)		
e. Total Free or Nominal Rate Distribution (Sum of 15d (1), (2), (3) and (4))		▲	49	55
f. Total Distribution (Sum of 15c and 15e)		▲	567	460
g. Copies not Distributed (See instructions to publishers #4 (page #3))		▲	468	390
h. Total (Sum of 15f and g)		▲	1035	850
i. Percent Paid (15c divided by 15f times 100)			91.36%	88.04%

16. Publication of Statement of Ownership
☐ If the publication is a general publication, publication of this statement is required. Will be printed in the **October 2011** issue of this publication.   Publication not required

17. Signature and Title of Editor, Publisher, Business Manager, or Owner

Amy S. Beacham – Senior Inventory Distribution Coordinator

Date
September 16, 2011

I certify that all information furnished on this form is true and complete. I understand that anyone who furnishes false or misleading information on this form or who omits material or information requested on the form may be subject to criminal sanctions (including fines and imprisonment) and/or civil sanctions (including civil penalties).

PS Form 3526, September 2007 (Page 2 of 3)

Moving?

Make sure your subscription moves with you!

To notify us of your new address, find your **Clinics Account Number** (located on your mailing label above your name), and contact customer service at:

Email: journalscustomerservice-usa@elsevier.com

800-654-2452 (subscribers in the U.S. & Canada)
314-447-8871 (subscribers outside of the U.S. & Canada)

Fax number: 314-447-8029

Elsevier Health Sciences Division
Subscription Customer Service
3251 Riverport Lane
Maryland Heights, MO 63043

Printed and bound by CPI Group (UK) Ltd, Croydon, CR0 4YY

03/10/2024

01040357-0013